HypnoVision

Also by Lisette Scholl

VISIONETICS:
The Holistic Way to Better Eyesight

LISETTE SCHOLL

Illustrations by Debbie Bartmasser

The *New* Natural Way

HypnoVision

to Vision Improvement

HENRY HOLT AND COMPANY
New York

Published by Henry Holt and Company, Inc.,
115 West 18th Street, New York, New York 10011.
Published in Canada by Fitzhenry & Whiteside Limited,
195 Allstate Parkway, Markham, Ontario L3R 4T8.

LIBRARY OF CONGRESS CATALOGING-IN-PUBLICATION DATA
Scholl, Lisette.
HypnoVision : the *new* natural way to vision improvement /
Lisette Scholl ; illustrations by Debbie Bartmasser.—1st ed.
p.   cm.
ISBN 0-8050-1133-1
1. Orthoptics.   2. Hypnotism—Therapeutic use.   3. Vision
disorders—Psychosomatic aspects.   4. Eye—Care and hygiene.
I. Title.
RE992.07S29   1990
617.7′55—dc20   89-29593
                                                      CIP

Henry Holt books are available at special discounts for
bulk purchases for sales promotions, premiums, fund-
raising, or educational use. Special editions or book ex-
cerpts can also be created to specification.

For details contact:

Special Sales Director
Henry Holt and Company, Inc.
115 West 18th Street
New York, New York 10011

First Edition

Designed by Kathryn Parise

Printed in the United States of America

Recognizing the importance of preserving the written word,
Henry Holt and Company, Inc., by policy, prints all
of its first editions on acid-free paper. ∞

1   3   5   7   9   10   8   6   4   2

To Brett,
for the clarity of his vision

Contents

List of Illustrations

Acknowledgments

I would like to thank the spirits of Dr. William H. Bates and Franz Anton Mesmer. Without their insights into the process of vision and the healing power of the mind, none of this would have been possible.

A heartfelt thanks to all my clients, for I learned as much from them as they did from me.

For their expertise and warmth I will always be indebted to Randall Churchill and Marleen Muldar, directors of the Hypnotherapy Training Institute.

Without the knowledge and compassion of Sandy Sidah this book could never have been written on a computer, and would most likely still be stuck in my typewriter.

But most of all, without the love and support of my husband, Brett Mitchell, I could never have found the time for this book. He cooked, he cleaned, he shopped. He did it all. And what's more important, he loved it. Whatta guy!

Introduction

Fifteen years ago I stumbled across Dr. William Bates's book *Better Eyesight Without Glasses* in a used-book store. Until that moment I had absolutely no idea that my vision could change for the better. It had been gradually deteriorating since I was thirteen, and no eye doctor had ever hinted that it would do anything except continue its decline into ever-increasing blurriness. I had once thought to ask what caused my nearsightedness, and I was informed that it was "hereditary bad luck." As I was adopted and knew nothing of my biological background, I couldn't argue with this information. When I finally met my birth parents five years ago, I was amused to discover that they both have exceptionally good eyesight, not even needing reading glasses as they age. But I was not surprised, because I had long since learned that the percentage of genetically caused vision problems is minuscule. Good vision is not something we are born with or without, it's a subconsciously learned skill that develops in accordance with our personality and our attitudes.

I learned from Dr. Bates that poor vision is caused by "mental tension." Vision is a function of the mind, not a mechanical process performed simply by the eyes. The more I read of Bates's theories, the more sound they seemed. Why should the eyes be the only organs in the body incapable of healing? That makes no sense, and rightly so, because it just isn't true. Convinced at both the intellectual and gut levels of the validity of Bates's findings that eyesight could be changed for the better, I embarked on what turned out to be a life-transforming odyssey into clear vision.

I began when I was twenty-nine with 20/100 vision in my left eye and 20/200 in my right eye. I had depended on glasses for seventeen years. Within six months after I began working to change my vision, the test results were 20/70 in my left eye and 20/100 in my right eye. Even more encouraging was the fact that these figures were for my worst visual days, and I often experienced bursts of crystal-clear vision. I was so excited about my visual changes that I began teaching others what I had learned. I worked alongside my students, and my vision continued to improve with theirs. But I also began to experience frustrations that interfered with the satisfactions.

Bates's book and all the others on the topic were filled with inspiring stories of complete visual recovery. But this wasn't happening for me or for the people I was working with. I began to get the feeling that there was a missing link somewhere. So I started looking beyond the traditional Bates method for answers to why our progress wasn't as quick and complete as we wanted. And I began finding out that vision was a holistic process—even more so than I had understood previously.

I found, for example, that posture has an impact on vision. So, being a yoga teacher, I added exercises to my regime that improved the circulation and energy flow into the eyes. Next I realized that the degree of tension in the shoulders, neck, and face that accompanies poor eyesight was not fully relaxed away by Bates's exercises. So I added massages to the program. Clear sight is also dependent on proper nutrients, so I emphasized a lighter, healthier diet. Then, while on a visit to Los Angeles, I looked in the phone book under "vision training." I found the names of some Bates teachers, but my eye was caught by a mysterious listing for something called the Radix Institute. Wondering what it could be, I made a call. Like my initial discovery of Bates's book, it was a life-changing experience.

Dr. Charles Kelley, the founder of the institute, had made such good improvements in his sight through the Bates method during the 1940s that he became one of its teachers. But, just as I had, he came to feel there was a missing link somewhere. He found it in the emotional release work of Wilhelm Reich. As I explored my own emotional depths through the neo-Reichian Radix work, I too came to realize that there was a lot more to the concept of "mental tension" than Bates had perceived. There were powerful emotions at the root of many visual dysfunctions. After I uncovered and released my own deep-seated feelings of fearfulness, my vision made another leap into further clarity.

Now I was seeing 20/50 in my left eye and 20/70 in the right one. I was comfortable and functional in most situations without glasses. I felt the improvement would continue, so it was time to share what I had learned with a larger audience. In 1978 my book *Visionetics: The Holistic Way to Better Eyesight* was published. Now as I continued teaching I also heard from readers who were making wonderful changes in their vision. But, alas, as time went on I began to realize that, again, changes weren't as great or as lasting as I had hoped they would be. This included my own vision, which stayed about the same except for those occasional delightful bursts of clarity. Finally I admitted to myself that there must be yet another missing link somewhere. Almost as if fate were guiding me, I began coming across magazine articles about the healing power of hypnosis. Blood pressure could be lowered, childbirth was painless, hemorrhaging could be stopped, circulation could be increased, and surgery could be performed without anesthesia. Even cancer patients deemed terminal had gone into remission. All of a sudden the eyes adjusting the necessary fraction of a millimeter for clear vision didn't seem like such an insurmountable task.

Off I went to the best school I could find to become a hypnotherapist. Not only did hypnosis supply this long-sought-after missing link for vision improvement, but it is also the most powerful transformational tool I have ever encountered. My own vision shot up to 20/40 on a bad day, and my whole life changed when I applied the principles of positive suggestion. Vision work is now one part of my larger hypnotherapy practice. My life is blessed with daily experiences of helping people fulfill their potentials not only visually but in every aspect of their lives. You will find this out for yourself as you begin tapping into the incredible power of your subconscious mind.

HypnoVision is a synthesis of the most important Bates exercises and the restructuring of your visual system through your subconscious. Depending on the type and degree of your visual problem, if you follow the programs that follow, you should expect to see dramatic and lasting changes in four to eight weeks. Perhaps even more important is that your inner vision of yourself will change just as much as your outer vision of the world around you.

Do remember, of course, that this book is not meant as a substitute for regular checkups and care by an eye doctor. Your sight is precious, and you most certainly want to utilize the power of science as well as your mind to maintain it.

1

HypnoVision

Until 1983 I used to spend a great deal of time and effort explaining that vision could change for the better. It was a big step for people to question the traditional optometric tenet that vision is fixed except for its ability to deteriorate. Then I came across a study that eliminated the need for my lengthy dissertations.

A Chicago psychiatrist working with patients with multiple personalities took them to an optometrist. While under hypnosis they were able to change personalities when asked to. The eye doctor examined the vision in each persona. He was astounded to discover that vision shifted right along with personality. For example, one nearsighted patient required a correction four times stronger in one identity than in another. Another patient had glaucoma in one personality but not in the others. Chris Sizemore, the subject of the book and movie *The Three Faces of Eve*, experienced different visual conditions in different personalities. Farsightedness, astigmatism, and color blindness also altered along with the personalities. These were not emotional interpretations of what was seen, there were actual measurable changes in the shape of the eyes and the pressure within them. Since that time other psychiatrists have continued to document this phenomenon. These findings completely shatter the

1

beliefs of the old school of vision. Not only is vision fluid and adaptable but also, under certain circumstances, changes can take place with lightning speed.

Naturally, it's not worth being a multiple personality so that you can experience visual changes this quickly. But work with these fragmented individuals has shed more light on the amazing complexities and capabilities of the human mind than any other endeavor had before. The most advanced computer is child's play compared to the inner workings of our mind. Even though we're just beginning to understand it, it's obvious that there is no force on earth more powerful than the human mind.

Our analytic, conscious mind serves us well in our daily thoughts and activities, but the real control tower is our subconscious mind. It not only regulates and controls all of our involuntary bodily functioning but it is also the seat of our emotions, beliefs, and habits. If you've ever tried to use conscious willpower to change a habit, such as smoking or overeating, you know firsthand just how ineffectual this level of thinking can be. Hypnosis accesses the subconscious, which is why it is so effective for everything from pain relief to weight control and vision improvement. If you can't change your belief system, you can't change its control of your habits and functions. I didn't understand the vital importance of subconscious beliefs until I studied hypnosis. Once I grasped this fact, I realized that this was a major cause of failure in the vision improvement methods I had been using. You can tell yourself a million times at the conscious level that you know you can make positive changes in your vision, but it's all to no avail if this message doesn't reach the subconscious level. What we get is what we really believe deep down inside.

As soon as I became certified as a hypnotherapist, I called my local students who had made positive changes but were not fully satisfied with their progress. The first one to make an appointment to explore hypnotic restructuring of her visual belief system was Sally, a twenty-four-year-old teacher who had worn glasses since she was twelve. Through the use of a pendulum, something you will be using later, we determined that indeed the only thing holding back her full recovery was her inner belief that it wasn't possible. After three sessions she discarded her glasses completely. On her birthday a few weeks later she passed the vision test for her driver's license. Then she went to the eye doctor, and it was confirmed that her vision was now 20/20.

Before you get too excited about the prospect of full and nearly immediate recovery of your clear vision, remember that Sally had already invested many months of time and effort in working with her vision. Also, her myopia (nearsightedness) was never very severe. When she began working with me, her vision was 20/60. But still, this gives you an idea of what a difference hypnosis can make.

And the difference can be even more profound at the emotional level. Behind the visual problems of some people lies a strong subconscious desire not to see clearly. As I discovered at the Radix Institute, I was one of these people. Sally was not, except for a brief period during her adolescence when she was embarrassed about the changes taking place in her body. She outgrew that stage, which shaped her vision, but glasses locked her into poor vision until she began vision work. Others of us had even more stress in our formative years. My own junior high years included my grandmother's broken back and then stroke, my mother's increasing alcoholism, more bitter dissension than usual between my divorced parents, and a move to a new town and school, in addition to the normal trauma of entering the teenage years. No wonder I didn't want to see clearly.

Shortly after Sally's wonderful breakthrough, I had a chance to work with someone whose visual dysfunction had had a far more traumatic beginning than mine. Jill, a forty-year-old nurse, had been nearsighted since she was seven. Her myopia was severe; she saw 20/200 in her left eye and 200/400 in her right eye. Her success at improving her vision had been slight. When I called her to see if she would like to try hypnosis, she was very hesitant. Finally she admitted that she was afraid of it because it might make her relive experiences she had never told me about. She had been sexually molested by her stepfather for much of her early life. I assured her that hypnosis provides a distancing and a buffer of emotional protection from memories of this sort. She thought about what I had said and later called for an appointment. Just before we began the

first session, she mentioned that while she had never before considered that the experience with her stepfather had an effect on her
vision, she did feel it was probably why she had never experienced
orgasm.

I took Jill back to that period of her life. While she was clearly
affected emotionally as she recounted what had happened, she was
removed from the scene, as if she were watching it on a movie
screen. Her subconscious confirmed that both her visual and sexual
problems were caused by the trauma of what had happened to her.
Through this session and several others I was able to convince her
subconscious that not all men were like her stepfather and that it was
okay to see clearly again. She called me the morning after she had
her first orgasm! Her eyesight also improved dramatically. Eventually, after we convinced her belief system that her sight was capable
of change, she no longer needed glasses except at work and while
driving.

I began working with new clients by addressing their belief systems
first. Then I had them perform all of the exercises I used with
Visionetics, either under hypnosis or with posthypnotic suggestions. Things went very well, but there were so many exercises to be
done that the process was still very time-consuming. So I began to
experiment with using fewer exercises. As time went on I found
myself paring the program down more and more and still achieving
greater success than ever before. It became another case of the
simpler the better. What appears here now as HypnoVision is the
result of a refinement procedure that boiled the techniques down to
those most effective in the shortest amount of time.

But I'm sure you are still wondering if you will really be able to
achieve 20/20 vision. My favorite title in hypnosis books is one about
the legendary Gil Boyne entitled *Miracles on Demand*. I've witnessed
Mr. Boyne perform some of these miracles. One, for example, is
known as the Case of the Chicago Stutterer, when he permanently
cured a man in his fifties of severe, lifelong stuttering in one dramatic session. I've also seen results in my own practice that truly
appear miraculous. But I can still claim only about a 30 percent rate

of total visual recovery with my clients. Yet that's nearly 29 percent more than before. And the number of people who become truly visually independent—needing, say, glasses only for night driving—has skyrocketed. The degree of your changes will depend on the length of time you have worn glasses, the extent of your problem, and how well you master the art of being a good hypnotic subject.

When people begin vision work, most tend to feel that there's no point to it unless they achieve 20/20 vision. Those optometrists who admit that natural techniques can improve eyesight also generally hold this attitude. Remember, though, that 20/20 is an arbitrary figure. It was the distance at which the average person can see a Snellen chart (the familiar eye chart) clearly. I say "was" because it is no longer the norm to see 20/20. A conservative estimate is that 60 percent of the population have visual defects of one sort or another. Technology, stress, and the pace of our lives have taken a terrific toll on our vision. So long as we make unreasonable demands on our vision, it is going to suffer.

Even though your vision still might need some occasional artificial help in stressful situations, that's no reason to sacrifice the ability to see unaided most of the time. Go for it. It's an experience that will transform you at every level of your being!

This book will guide you through every phase of becoming your own hypnotist and vision teacher. I have duplicated what I do in my practice as accurately as possible. Self-hypnosis and the vision exercises are fun and easy to master. You'll learn the dynamics of your own vision problem and be able to choose and tailor the program that best suits your needs. You'll gain not only clearer vision but also a deeper understanding of your own personal power and your innate ability to create your own positive reality.

It's an adventure of self-discovery and change. Welcome! This is a journey into the most powerful force in the universe, the human mind, your mind.

Your journey begins with knowledge. The first five chapters (and the introductory material in Chapter 6) of this book supply information that is vital to the success of the programs that follow. Don't just skim over the material, study it. In fact, as you become involved in the specific program designed to change your visual dysfunction, you may find it very useful to refer now and then to the introductory material so that you always understand just what it is you are trying to accomplish. This will be particularly true if you are not nearsighted (myopic) or farsighted (presbyopic). Since these are the two most prevalent visual conditions, the programs for them are detailed completely (Chapters 6 and 7). The other programs are based on these two, and on the myopia program in particular. In the chapter or section on your own dysfunction you will be directed to make changes in these core programs to create one tailored for your particular needs. If you take the time to absorb the basic facts about your vision, you'll find it a simple matter to make the necessary changes. Vision is a fascinating process, and I'm sure you'll enjoy learning about it as much as changing it.

2

How We See

Only 10 percent of the visual process occurs in the eyes. The other 90 percent is a function of the optic center of the brain, which is located at the base of the skull in the *occipital lobe*. It is part of the subconscious, which regulates and controls all of our involuntary functions. The eyes record images under the direction of the brain and then send these bits of visual information to the brain to be interpreted into what we actually see. The occipital lobe interacts with all the other portions of the brain. We are holistic organisms in which every part is influenced by every other part. Knowing this, you can begin to get an idea of just how complex sight is.

Even though it's your mind that does the seeing, we'll begin exploring how we see by starting with the front surface of the eye and working our way back to the control tower. The changes you will experience will manifest in your eyes themselves, so it's the best place to start.

Actually, we first have to start with light. Without light there is no sight, for what we perceive as a visual image is the reflection of light off the object we are observing. Light contains all the colors of the spectrum. Objects absorb certain colors and reflect others. What we see are the colors that are rejected by the object. What we see as a

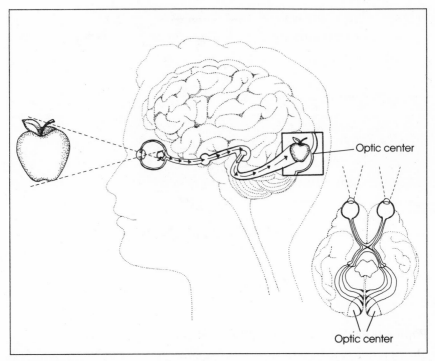

The Visual Process

red apple, for example, is one that has absorbed all the colors except red. It's almost as if we see what is left over. These reflected light waves pass through various layers of the eye and come to rest on its back surface, a photosensitive layer called the *retina*—ideally, that is. The light waves must be bent at just the right angle for them to land directly on the retina. This proper bending depends on each part of the eye doing its part of the procedure.

Cornea

The clear front surface of your eye is the *cornea*. It is made up of living cells that receive nourishment through the *aqueous humor* behind it. As you can see in the illustrations of the ideal eye, a properly shaped cornea is smooth and gently rounded. From the outside it is kept clean and moist and is protected by our eyelids. Our blinking reflex spreads the fluid secreted by our tear ducts over the cornea and responds to threats of penetration by foreign objects.

Aqueous Humor

After it is past the cornea, the light continues on through the aqueous humor. This watery fluid fills the anterior chamber of the eye and is secreted into and drained out of this chamber every four hours through a tiny opening known as the *canal of Schlemm*. The canal is a tube within the wall of the eye that empties the aqueous humor into one side of the anterior chamber and then drains it back out on the other side. The aqueous humor brings nourishment to the cornea and maintains the pressure necessary to sustain the cornea's curvature.

Pupil and Iris

The *pupil* is the black opening in the center of the eye, and the *iris* is the colored area around it. The muscles of the iris regulate the

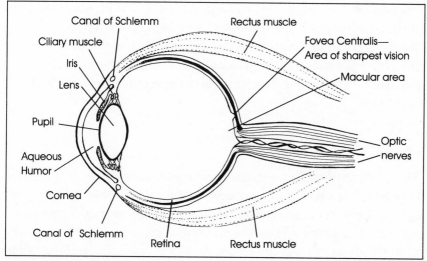

Cross Section of the Human Eye

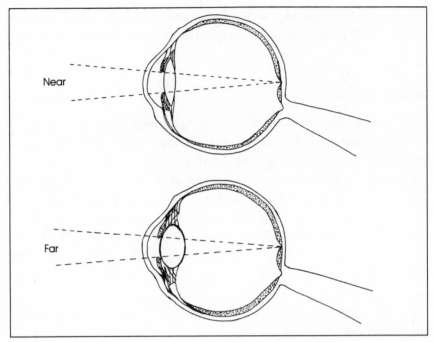

Lens Accommodation

amount of light entering the eye. If the light is very bright the muscles narrow in protection, and in dimness they expand to take advantage of what light is available. This helps in focusing the light directly on the retina. In addition, pupil size changes according to different emotional responses. When we look at something pleasurable, for example, such as parents observing a newborn, there is a widening of the pupil. Fear can also expand the pupil, while anger narrows it.

Lens and Ciliary Muscles

The single biggest factor in the bending of incoming light is the *lens.* It begins as a single cell, and new layers are added as we grow and age. It looks very much like an onion and is encased in an outer capsule. The shape of the lens changes according to how far we are from the object of our attention. As you can see in the illustration, the lens has a round, convex shape for distance and changes into a flatter, more concave shape when we focus close up. This process of shifting is known as *accommodation*. But the lens does not do this by itself. A set of tiny muscles, the *ciliary muscles,* attached to each side of the lens performs the actual shifting, and the lens simply stretches in the direction it is pulled by these muscles. The muscles are relaxed when we look out into the distance, and they tighten up to bring our lenses into the flatter shape for nearpoint focusing.

Extraocular Muscles

Outside the eyeball are two sets of muscles that control the balancing and movement of the eyes, the *recti* and the *oblique.* Dr. Bates concluded that these muscles, as opposed to the lens and ciliary muscles, performed the function of accommodation. He felt that the recti muscles pulled the eye into a shorter shape for distance viewing and that the oblique muscles squeezed the eye into a longer shape for close work. According to Bates, chronic tension in these muscles inhibited the eyes from being able to adjust their focus. The opto-

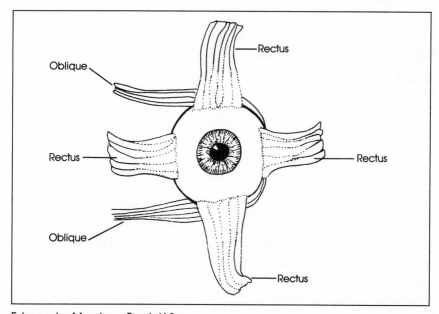

Extraocular Muscles—Frontal View

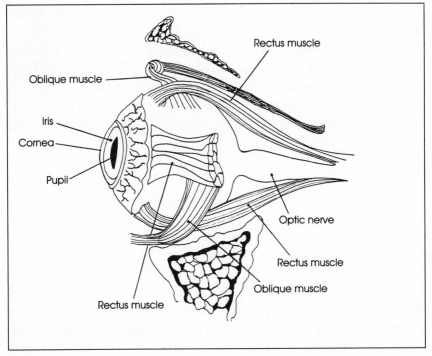

Parts of the Eye

metric community stuck to its theory of lens accommodation by the ciliary muscles, and the issue has remained in hot dispute ever since. My own conclusion is that the lens does the focusing, but emotional tension manifests itself in the extraocular muscles and forces the eyes out of their proper shape.

Vitreous Humor

After the light passes through the lens, it continues its journey through the *vitreous humor.* This jellylike substance supports the shape of the eye and helps nourish the retina. Unlike the aqueous humor, this fluid is never changed or replenished. Should an injury occur that allowed the vitreous humor to leak out, the eye would be unable to regain its shape.

Retina

Finally the light now falls on its destination, the *retina*. This is an extraordinarily complex, ten-layered tissue of brain cells. The layer in charge of recording the information carried by the light is made of nerve cells known as *rods* and *cones*. It is also bathed in a chemical called *rhodopsin,* or visual purple, which stimulates the rods and cones to accept the incoming light. The rods occur toward the outer edges of the retina, and the cones are concentrated toward the center. The rods record black and white and large shapes and are responsible for our peripheral vision. The cones perceive color and detail. The highest concentration of these nerve cells is in the center of the retina in a tiny spot known as the *macula.* In the center of the macula, the *fovea centralis,* they are even more densely packed together. This is the point of our clearest and most detailed vision. The light-sensitive rods and cones vibrate constantly as they pick up the incoming bits of visual information.

It is interesting to note that images are recorded upside down on the retina. As the brain interprets these images, it turns them right side up. We don't know why this happens, but a research experiment on this phenomenon showed just how flexible the visual system can be. A man was fitted with prism lenses that turned the images over. For about a week he viewed the world as upside down. By that time the brain was fed up with this disorienting view, so it made the necessary adjustments and began interpreting the images as right side up again. As you progress through the HypnoVision program, you'll be asking the optic center of your brain to make a few small adjustments, so remember just how flexible it can be!

Another point worth mentioning here is that approximately 20 percent of retinal functioning has nothing to do with sight. The colors of the light spectrum literally feed our bodies. Our master glands, the pituitary and pineal, are stimulated and regulated by light. Conditions from arthritis to infertility to mood swings are all affected by the type and degree of light we are exposed to. We need light for life as well as for sight.

Optic Nerves

Our eyes are connected to our brain by the *optic nerves*. They are made up of a bundle of nerves that number over a million. While we are developing in the womb, our eyes grow outward from the brain itself into their sockets. The optic nerves become the conduit along which messages pass from the retina to the brain. They are coated with a protective layer of insulation called *myelin*. This coating is not completed until infants are ten to twelve weeks old, which is part of the reason it takes their vision so long to be functional. The optic nerves cross in the center of our brain, where they exchange visual input from each eye so that we get a coherent picture.

The Brain

Light waves transformed into electrical impulses travel down the optic nerves to the brain, and it is here that the image is interpreted into what we actually see. This miraculous biocomputer sorts through all the bits of visual information it has received and constructs them into a coherent picture. The optic center of the brain is the control tower of the eye's functioning as well as the receiver of the images. It directs the blinking, moving, and focusing of our eyes through a constant barrage of finely coordinated signals. This is why a blow to the back of the head can have such an impact on vision. My dog, for example, was hit by a car when he was a puppy, suffering a blow to the back of the head, and his pupils became frozen in the wide-open position. Being a dog, he was unable to reeducate his brain to correct the signal and was essentially blind. But barring the most severe of injuries or disease, we humans can reeducate the optic center of our brain to both send and receive clearer signals. Like the researcher with the prism glasses, we can change and adapt to our visual world. And, because vision is one of the functions of the subconscious portion of the mind, you will find that hypnosis is the ideal tool for accessing and making changes in this area.

3

Why We Don't See Clearly

You've seen how the optimal eye works under perfect conditions, so let's move on to reality. The bottom line is that approximately 60 percent of the population suffers from some sort of visual dysfunction. Clear sight has become an aberration rather than the norm. The progressives in the optometric field attribute this development to the visual stresses and strains of modern society, such as being indoors, reading, and television watching. The old guard still insist that heredity is the cause of poor vision, even though study after study has proved otherwise. The real answer lies in an expansion of the theory supported by the progressive optometrists.

It is true that we still have cavemen's eyes but are asking them to operate in a world different from the one for which they were created. The general population does a lot more close work than ever before. However, half the caveperson population were women, and they used their eyes for a lot of close work. There is a tendency to talk about the eyes of hunters scanning the horizon for game, but we should not forget that the women were home cooking, sewing, and caring for babies. Even planting and harvesting crops involved mostly near vision. Thus cavepeople used their eyes in ways similar to those of modern people, yet their vision didn't suffer.

It is also the emotional complexity of our world today, rather than just its books and tools, that has created the visual responses so many of us suffer from. Think about nearsightedness as a pulling in from, a shutting out of events we'd rather not be exposed to, much less see. Now think about world conditions—everything from the possibility of nuclear holocaust to the greenhouse effect to the rising rate of rapes and child molestations. Whew. We are to be commended on our adaptability, our ability to live in this way at all rather than just running off to the mountains and hiding out in a cave. No wonder 40 percent of the population is nearsighted. And on top of that we have all the personal traumas of our individual lives. We have a lot to contend with, and it's not difficult to believe that this barrage of influences would alter our power of perception.

Keeping all this in mind, we'll go back through the eye and visual system again. This time you'll learn just how each part can be influenced by how we perceive reality, and how our vision is affected.

Cornea

If your cornea is damaged or misshapen you won't see clearly, even if everything else is in perfect working order. Injuries and certain diseases can scar this delicate tissue. Light will reflect off these scars in a diffuse manner and fail to come to rest on the detail-seeking macula, with the result being blurred vision. Years ago I caught an eye infection known as conjunctivitis, your common garden-variety "pink eye," which then developed into herpes on my cornea after an eye doctor gave me inappropriate medication. By the time I was rushed, in excruciating pain, to another doctor, severe ulcerations had formed. For a while it looked as if my cornea might be permanently scarred. I was lucky, however, and the ulcers gradually healed. But in the meantime I found out what it was like to have vision far more blurry than I had ever experienced. Strangely, this event turned out to be a blessing that changed my life. I became unable to wear contact lenses, as they irritated my eyes and caused the herpes to recur. This left me with my glasses, which I hated. Then I found Dr. Bates's book, and the rest, as they say, is history. Had I been able to tolerate contacts, I might never have had any interest in natural methods of vision improvement. How we live and learn and grow!

Fortunately, most people don't encounter the problem of injury or disease to their corneas. However, there is one common, chronic problem that is close to being an injury. Many people, especially *myopes* (nearsighted people) have such tension in their eyelids that the blinking reflex is inhibited. To see clearly, the cornea must be moist. Teaching students to remember to blink often enough at the conscious level so that the blinking habit once again became regular and spontaneous was extremely tedious work, and often the students never developed the habit. Because hypnosis goes directly to the subconscious control of the blinking reflex, this is no longer a problem.

A misshapen cornea is far more common than a damaged one. An imbalanced pull by the extraocular muscles results in a warping of the cornea. Instead of one clear image there is an overlapping or

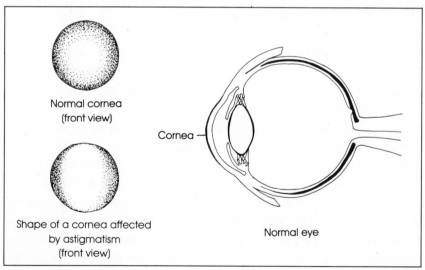

Normal cornea
(front view)

Cornea —

Shape of a cornea affected
by astigmatism
(front view)

Normal eye

Astigmatism

distortion of the images, as opposed to or in addition to a general softness of the image. This is what's known as *astigmatism*. It can occur for both physical and emotional reasons.

I can often tell if someone has astigmatism just by observing him or her. The imbalance in the eye muscles is usually a reflection of an imbalance in the rest of the body as well. If you have astigmatism, look in the mirror. Does your head tilt a bit to one side? Is one shoulder higher than the other? Does one hip rotate out farther than the other? If you look noticeably lopsided, you may want to add massage, bodywork or chiropractic, or a posture-balancing exercise routine such as yoga, all discussed later, to the Hypno-Vision program.

Poor reading habits, especially during the formative years, can also create astigmatism. Lying on your side while reading can pull the eye muscles out of balance. Holding the book off to one side can have the same effect. If this applies to you, you'll find that the combination of gentle Bates exercises and hypnotic suggestions in this book will ease your eyes back into alignment.

Still another physical cause of astigmatism is poor development of early motor skills and hand/eye coordination. In countries in which the young are swaddled, including some American Indian tribes, surveys of vision problems have turned up a correlation with astigmatism. It also shows up in many children who skipped much of their crawling phase and went right on to walking. Beyond these physical factors there are also emotional ones. Immigrants beginning the process of acculturation often develop astigmatism. So do people exposed to other kinds of confusing inputs, such as being shuttled between divorced parents or living with an alcoholic parent who constantly sends out mixed messages.

Confusion is the operative term here. This emotional response pattern quite literally throws the eyes off balance. Again, the way we see the world is reflected in our vision. With hypnotic uncovering and suggestion and gentle smoothing exercises, astigmatic eyes respond quite well. You can tell if you have astigmatism by looking at the illustration with the circles on the next page—without your glasses, of course! Even if you know there is a correction for astigmatism in your prescription, you'll find it interesting to observe the

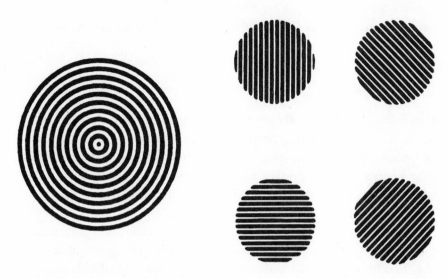

Astigmatism Evaluation Chart

circles, because the dark area reflects the space on your cornea where warping exists. Look at the four circles with the lines across them. If one is darker than the rest, you have astigmatism. It is the same with the concentric circles. There's a warp in your cornea if a pie-shaped section seems to stand out as different. You can refer to these circles as you progress through the program, and you'll see your progress in black and white.

Aqueous Humor

Glaucoma is most often caused when a malfunction of the canal of Schlemm stops the fluid from the anterior chamber from draining out every four hours. When the aqueous humor can't get back out, pressure builds up inside the eye. Eventually this pressure affects the nerves of the retina. First the peripheral vision is affected, and then later the central, or detail, vision is also damaged. The result can be blindness.

The early detection of glaucoma is one of the best reasons for regular optometric checkups. Medication can usually control the problem, and hypnosis and the relaxation exercises can enhance its performance.

Iris and Pupil

Our iris muscles expand or contract our pupils to regulate incoming light. With age these muscles do not expand quite as much as would be optimal to focus up close. If you are *presbyopic,* the farsightedness that begins sometime after forty, you've noticed that you can see print better in bright light. The extra illumination makes up for the narrowness of the pupil.

Myopia, nearsightedness, on the other hand, is often accompanied by pupils that do not contract enough when looking out into the distance. The light waves are diffused instead of being aimed directly at the retina. If a myope stands next to someone with clear distance vision, the pupilar difference between their eyes can actually be seen. Nearsighted people with overwidening of the pupils are often those who have responded with fear to the circumstances of their lives. Pupils widen when we are fearful, and they stay that way if the response continues for an extended period of time. Pupil size is just a small portion of what makes up myopia, but like the other components it responds positively to the HypnoVision program.

Lens and Ciliary Muscles

To continue seeing clearly when we shift our focus in and out, the lens must change shape. If it doesn't change enough the image will fall in front of or behind the retina. Myopia occurs if the image falls in front of the retina. Both types of farsightedness, presbyopia, already mentioned, and *hyperopia* (the type that starts at an early age), occur when the lens focuses the image behind the retina.

In the next section you will see that the extraocular muscles contribute to myopia and hyperopia, but the lens also plays a powerful role. When I first began working with my vision, Bates's conclusion that the extraocular muscles were the cause of my nearsightedness made sense to me. Then I had occasion to discover truth in the optometric view of the lens being at fault.

I had gone to the eye doctor for a reduction in my prescription, and he convinced me to try bifocal lenses as well. Instead of the single-prescription lens doing all the focusing work for me, my ciliary muscles were now forced to work too, by loosening and tightening their pull on my lenses when I changed the distance of my focus. I experienced dizziness and discomfort for a while, but it wasn't long before there was a 20 percent improvement in my distance vision. This was before I had done any of the Bates exercises, so the changes couldn't have come from anything else. To make further progress I still had to do a lot more work on my own, but I now knew that the optometric viewpoint had validity. Clearly, the shape of both the eye and the lens were involved.

Too much focusing at close range, such as reading or working on a computer, creates spasm in the ciliary muscles that control the movement of the lens. They simply won't let go so the lens can spring into the convex shape for distance vision. In the Hypno-Vision program for myopia, you'll be getting those muscles to relax when you shift your focus out into the distance. If you feel that it was simply too much close work that caused your myopia, this relaxing will be a primary aid to regaining your overall clear sight.

If you are presbyopic you'll be toning the ciliary muscles as well as getting circulation into the lenses so that they are flexible again. If you are hyperopic you'll be concentrating on teaching those muscles to tighten up properly to move the lenses. Hyperopic lenses lack flexibility but do not suffer from the poor circulation that accompanies presbyopia. If you are a "presbee," you can start thinking right now if you can make life-style changes that will also increase the circulation into your lenses. If you developed this condition before you were forty-five, chances are you are either very sedentary or a smoker. Smoking cuts down drastically on circulation, particularly to delicate areas like the eyes. Smokers generally begin becoming presbyopic ten years earlier than other people. Yet another good reason to give it up!

Lack of moisture and nutrients to the lenses can also be instrumental in the formation of *cataracts*. "Cataract" comes from the Latin word for waterfall, and trying to see through one is very much like trying to look through a veil of water. But cataracts are really opacities in the lenses. Sediment forms as the lenses are robbed of circulation and nutrients, and the light cannot pass through on its way to the retina.

Some cases of cataracts seemed to be linked to excessive heat and glare, as there is a high incidence among fishermen and steelworkers stationed near furnaces. Intense light and heat dry out the eye's moisture and nutrients. However, the majority of cases are more clearly related to lack of circulation and, as a result, lack of nutrients. Everything coming into the eyes has to be so finely filtered that circulation is easily obstructed. Smoking, drinking, lack of exercise, and a variety of prescription drugs, especially those in the cortisone family, both sap nutrients and cut off circulation. In the section on vitamins (page 29) you'll find information on what to add to your diet and exercise regime. While advanced cases of cataracts are probably candidates for the surgical removal of the lens and implantation of an artificial one, early cases respond well to hypnosis and the relaxation exercises that open circulation. In fact, several of my elderly clients with advanced cataracts but an aversion to any kind of surgical procedures used the HypnoVision program in addition to diet and exercise programs (one chose swimming and the other went with yoga), and their cataracts cleared to the point where they could get by comfortably with just a mild prescription for glasses.

Extraocular Muscles

As I've already mentioned, Dr. Bates was certain that accommodation was achieved by the extraocular muscles changing the shape of the eye. The optometric viewpoint is that these muscles simply balance and turn the eyes. I feel extraocular muscles may have some role in accommodation, but I agree with the traditionalists that the lens is primary in accommodation. Even though Dr. Bates and I disagree on the extent of the focusing power of these muscles, we fully concur that tension in them results in myopia, hyperopia, astigmatism, and *strabismus* (eyes that turn either in or out).

In myopia, except for mild cases where the ciliary muscles alone

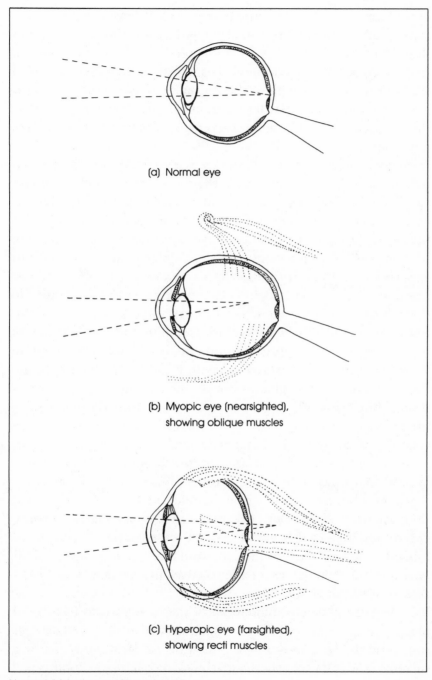

(a) Normal eye

(b) Myopic eye (nearsighted),
showing oblique muscles

(c) Hyperopic eye (farsighted),
showing recti muscles

Normal, Myopic, and Hyperopic Eyes

are at fault, the oblique muscles that encircle the eye are so tight that the eyeball is squeezed into an elongated shape, and the image falls short of the retina. In hyperopia, the recti muscles stretching from front to back are in a cramped spasm that shortens the eyeball so that the image falls behind the retina. If only one of the rectus muscles is tight, the eye will turn in or out. An imbalanced pull by these muscles will result in the warping of the cornea that produces astigmatism.

Wilhelm Reich's theory of "muscular armoring" is the best explanation for the extreme tension in the extraocular muscles. Varying emotional reactions result in the body trying to protect the mind by building barriers to feeling. The emotions become immobilized inside the frozen bands of muscles. We don't feel the pain anymore, but neither do we have the good feelings that we were meant to experience as well. In addition to remaining cut off from our emotions, we develop physical problems due to tension—everything from lower back pain to heart attacks to poor eyesight. Reich developed a therapy based on breathing that restored energy to the muscles while freeing both them and the blocked emotions. Then these emotions can be dealt with from the healthier perspective of the present. Reichian work can be lengthy and emotionally trying, but by combining the basic theory with the gentlest of breathing exercises and hypnotic suggestion, I have used it successfully in my hypnotherapy practice.

Because of some of the rather traumatic situations in my background that contributed to my own myopia, I originally assumed that everyone else who was nearsighted had also experienced the same intensity of fear. But I discovered that while some had experienced even greater degrees of fearfulness, most people simply exhibited a minor but continual avoidance of looking at their environment. Where fear is the operative emotion behind a myopia case, it need not be intense.

The same is true of hyperopia, which is related to feelings of blocked anger. The desire to avoid irritation as well as actual anger can cause the recti muscles to tighten down. Strabismus can be a turning away from, as opposed to a blocking out of, irritation as well as anger. And so it is with astigmatism, where the confusion may also be minor but habitual enough to lock into a pattern.

Most people are essentially free from the emotional reactions that originally shaped their visual dysfunction, but glasses and habit have maintained the condition. However, if the straightforward restructuring and healing of your visual system does not bring about the changes you desire, you will have the opportunity to deal with your past in Chapter 12, "Regression." But, again, the odds are that reeducating your eye/brain responses will be all the work you will need.

Vitreous Humor

For the vast majority of us light passes unimpeded through the vitreous humor on its way to the retina. However, in a few people bits of the vitreous humor coagulate into small particles. These are called *floaters* and are quite literally seen as little black specks or squiggles floating through the visual image. They are harmless but quite annoying. Optometry has no way of treating this condition, and people are simply advised to ignore floaters. This can be akin to telling someone not to think about pink elephants. Fortunately, massage, diet, and relaxation along with hypnotic suggestions can increase circulation in the vitreous humor so dramatically that these particles break up and the floaters disappear.

Retina

The common errors of refraction from which most of us suffer do not involve malfunctioning within the retina. Many more serious problems, however, are related to the functioning of this light-sensitive area.

Night blindness is common in small degrees to most of us, but severe cases of it seriously hamper an individual's ability to function at all in the dark. The visual purple that stimulates the rods and cones to do their job is particularly important for night vision. It depends on adequate quantities of vitamin A to stay in top working order. If there is a deficiency of this vitamin, the retina becomes less sensitive to incoming light and is unable to adjust to changes in the amount of illumination. Hypnotic suggestion combined with dietary changes can make a world of difference.

Amblyopia, or lazy-eye blindness, occurs when the nerves in one retina shut down. The apparatus is there, but it ceases to function as it should. There is no officially known cause for amblyopia, but the problem is really in the brain, which stops sending the appropriate signals. Many cases of amblyopia occur in conjunction with an eye that turns in or out. The brain quickly tires of trying to interpret the two very different images being sent to it and turns one of them off. With only one eye working, there is a significant loss of depth perception.

Our eyes reflect the two sides of our brain. The right side is associated with the dominant, aggressive, analytical part of our thinking. The left side governs our creative, nurturing, feeling aspects. You can also stretch these analogies to include father with the right side and mother with the left. Many people who suffer from amblyopia confirm that the eye that quit working relates to their emotional makeup and, often, with unresolved conflicts with mother or father figures. Acknowledging this can be beneficial. One woman in her early twenties whom I regressed back to childhood recalled previously blocked-out instances when she had rebuffed sexual advances from her alcoholic father. She had reacted with anger rather than fear, but she had turned away from and shut out the response rather than confront her father. After she remembered the events from her childhood, the nerves in her right eye began to function again almost immediately. This gave her temporarily overlapping images, but her eyes just as quickly responded to relaxation and retraining through exercises and more hypnosis. She soon saw clear single images of the world around her. Her youth enabled this quick recovery—the nerves had not been shut down so long that they couldn't reactivate.

A very dangerous condition known as *detached retina* occurs when the retina tears away from the lining of the eye. It happens most often when an individual with a high degree of myopia, whose retina is already stretched very thin due to the elongation of the eyeball, receives a blow to the head. This can result in blindness and should receive immediate medical attention. I never work with persons with detached retinas unless they are also under a doctor's care. Relaxation and hypnosis can aid in the healing process but are best used in conjunction with laser treatment, a scientific development that has saved the sight of many thousands of people.

If the rods in the retina do not function properly, we lose our peripheral and night vision. The condition known as *retinitis pigmentosa,* or tunnel vision, is the most extreme of these cases. Nourishment and stimulation to the rods is lacking, apparently due to genetic problems (one of the very few eye conditions that is hereditary), and the person quite literally sees as if through a black, narrow tunnel. Coupled with medical care, HypnoVision can be helpful in providing relaxation and stimulation to the rods and teaches habits of vision that expand the visual field.

If the cones malfunction we lose our central vision, and this is called *macular degeneration.* This happens to some people when age and lack of circulation cut off nutrients to the cones. Again, medical attention is in order, but I have witnessed many people reactivate their detailed vision through relaxation, exercise, vitamins, and powerful hypnotic suggestion. Sometimes this loss of central vision occurs in young people, and while it, too, may be primarily genetic in origin, I have worked with some people who concluded that the cause was emotional. One young man, for example, after I regressed him to his childhood, had vivid memories of the constant expression of hatred in his father's eyes. He realized that he had simply not wanted to see this central detail in his life. He blocked it out successfully but, of course, sacrificed his entire capacity for central vision at the same time. By coming to grips with these feelings and retraining his visual attitude, he was able to regain much of his detailed sight.

Optic Nerve

For the vast majority of us, the optic nerves perform their job of carrying messages back and forth between the eyes and the brain quite well. In some severe cases of glaucoma, the pressure caused by this disease can destroy the optic nerves. But the most common disorder is *tobacco amblyopia*. Smoking destroys the vitamin B12 necessary to maintain the insulative coating of myelin around the optic nerve. The result is a dimming of vision, but it is usually reversed when cigarettes are given up.

The Brain

Finally we're back to the brain, that wonderful biocomputer that both instructs the eyes in their functioning and interprets all those bits of visual information into the images we see. The optic portion of the brain interacts with the rest of our mind, and our sight is influenced by everything around us and our reaction to our environment. The way we see is very much a reflection of our individual perceptions and responses.

The HypnoVision approach to understanding and healing vision utilizes direct contact with this control tower of sight more than any other program I know of. Once the brain understands exactly what changes you desire, it will, with its incomparable power, execute your commands. It can direct physiological change, send better instructions to your eyes, and be trained to interpret more clearly the images sent to it. The interpreting will probably improve first. This often results in a somewhat amusing response from eye doctors. When my clients first go in to have their prescriptions reduced, they are often told that they shouldn't pay any attention to the increases in their vision because it is merely the result of improved interpretation. Merely? Clarity is clarity, and to discount this marvelous ability of the brain to make up for deficiencies in the eyes is ludicrous! And yet interpretation is just the beginning, and organic changes soon follow.

Other Factors

Illness when accompanied by a high fever can damage the eyes, especially in those already nearsighted. What our grandmothers told us about not reading when we were sick is not an old wives' tale. The eye is softened when fever is present, and therefore it is easily pushed more out of shape by the pressure created when our lenses contract to read print. If the reading is done with glasses meant for distance, the lens has to accommodate twice as much as without those glasses. This adds even more pressure inside the eye. If you are myopic, don't read with your glasses on if you can avoid it, especially when you are sick. A bifocal lens is another alternative, as this allows the lens to change its shape.

The effect illness can have on vision is illustrated by the experience I had with Rick, a thirty-year-old construction worker. He was myopic enough to need glasses when he worked, but he hated them because they were constantly slipping down his nose on hot days when he began to sweat. He was an outgoing, athletic man with no reasons we could determine for his myopia. He was not much of a reader nor had there been any emotional upheavals in his upbringing. Only after those sessions that involved the healing visualizations did he see better. Finally he just happened to mention that the only novel he remembered reading that wasn't required in school was Jack London's *The Call of the Wild* when he was sick with the measles. With that information we simply concentrated on the healing visualization. After several months his myopia was reduced to the point where he felt comfortable working without wearing glasses.

Vitamins are essential to the proper functioning of our eyes. Because nutrients are so finely filtered by the time they reach our eyes, any depletion in them has a particularly strong impact on our vision. As you read through the following information on vitamins, consider your diet and decide if it would benefit you to make some changes or additions to the way you now eat.

Let's do this alphabetically, beginning with the vitamin you've always heard was good for your vision. A deficiency of *vitamin A* can result in night blindness and a dried-out cornea. Severe cases of dry cornea can lead to blindness, and lesser degrees of dryness are not only uncomfortable but also make the eye susceptible to conjunctivitis, a nasty inflammation that itches and burns. Vitamin A is in great demand by the eyes and is eaten up by everything from night driving, exposure to excessive heat and glare, and nicotine and alcohol to flickering fluorescent lights, television, and video display terminals. The best way to replenish your supply of vitamin A is to consume copious amounts of those marvelous orange and leafy dark green vegetables you've been hearing about that also fend off cancer. If you take supplements, make sure they are the water-soluble beta carotene type that cannot result in an overdose.

All the *B vitamins* are necessary for the visual system to function well. *Thiamin,* vitamin B1, keeps the eye muscles working smoothly, and a severe lack of it has been linked to paralysis of these muscles. *Riboflavin,* B2, must be present or the eyes will become unduly sensitive to light, constantly fatigued, burning and bloodshot, and unable to see clearly in the twilight hours. B2 also appears to play a role in the circulation of nutrients to the lenses as a deficiency usually shows up in cataract patients. *B6* is important for the emotional stability that can insure a healthy reaction to life's trials and tribulations. *B12* also soothes our emotions, and it is the vitamin sapped by smoking, which results in tobacco amblyopia. A lack of *B15* shows up in individuals who suffer from cataracts and glaucoma. All of the B vitamins are eaten up by stress, alcohol, tobacco, sugar, and caffeine. The best sources of them are those leafy dark greens, Brewer's yeast, grains, eggs, meat, and nuts and seeds, especially sunflower seeds. If you take supplements make sure you get the whole family of Bs, as they need each other to be fully absorbed by your body.

Like vitamin A, *vitamin C* is another substance that not only aids vision but also fights everything from the common cold to cancer. To be fully effective vitamin C must contain both *ascorbic acid* and *bioflavinoids.* Man-made ascorbic acid is economical, but it appears that we also need the organic compounds found in the bioflavinoids. They are vital to circulation within the eyes, and high concentrations of them are found in healthy lenses. Vitamin C, especially that in the bioflavonoid *rutin,* is also important for the maintenance of capillary strength within the eyes. In addition, vitamin C has an antibiotic effect on corneal ulcers. Smoking destroys this vitamin, as do stress and a number of drugs, including antibiotics and cortisone. Citrus fruits, melons, and tomatoes are good sources of vitamin C. If you like to grow sprouts to garnish your salads, try buckwheat—it's one of the very best sources of rutin.

Vitamin D and *calcium* go hand in hand. They need each other in order for our bodies to absorb them, and in nature they often occur in conjunction with vitamin A. Myopes have low levels of calcium within their eyes. Several controlled studies found that high doses of calcium had a positive effect on myopia, detached retina, and glaucoma. With myopia it appears that calcium dehydrates the fluid within the eye, thus making the eyeball shorter. Sugar, especially in carbonated drinks, seems to be the major culprit in eyes so waterlogged that they stretch into the elongated, myopic shape. These eyes shrink back into a more round shape when calcium is present. The doses of calcium that were taken in these studies would be unsafe without medical supervision, but we need calcium-rich foods for the health of both the inside of our eyes and the eye muscles. Dairy products and those leafy dark greens, provided they are cooked, supply good amounts of calcium. Vitamin D is added to most milk, but the most natural source of it is sunlight, in moderate amounts, of course. Later you will learn a Bates exercise called Sunning that will allow you to absorb vitamin D while also relaxing your eyes and improving the circulation into them.

Vitamin E enables the bloodstream to carry necessary oxygen and nutrients to all parts of the body, and the eyes are no exception. This youth-enhancing substance is particularly important for maintaining the elasticity of the eye muscles and the lens. Doctors treating young myopes with vitamin E found that their lenses could spring back more readily into the convex shape for distance viewing if this vitamin was in good supply. In older people the lenses are kept clear as well as flexible when plenty of vitamin E is available. Pollutants, especially smog and smoke, drain away this vitamin, but those leafy dark greens will replenish it. Supplements are also handy, and you can gradually work up to 1,200 units a day.

Vitamins have a symbiotic relationship with each other. We need the full range if we are to assimilate them. There's no real substitute for the ideal balanced diet, but in this day and age it's hard to achieve. Between the stress of modern life and the depletions of the soil, to say nothing of pesticides and herbicides, we need all the help we can get. Taken sensibly, supplements can help your general health as well as your vision.

I've touched on the subject of *posture* already, but it is important enough to expand upon. It can be a powerful influence on conditions besides astigmatism, myopia in particular. Muscle imbalances and tension throughout the body not only create a lopsided pull on the eye muscles but also cut off circulation and energy needed by the visual system. Just as I can often spot people with astigmatism, I can also usually identify myopes even when they are wearing contact lenses or going without their glasses. Above tense shoulders the neck protrudes forward instead of straight up, and the chin juts out. There is also noticeable tension in the jaws of most nearsighted people. Whenever the base of the skull is compressed against the neck, the flow of circulation into the optic center of the brain diminishes. This postural stance also creates facial tension around the eyes as well as a corresponding tightness in the extraocular muscles. Reversing this is not just a simple matter of lifting your head up straighter, though it is certainly helpful. However, no area of the spine is independent of the rest. With myopes, for example, the jutting forward of the chin is usually accompanied by locked, hyperextended knees and hips that tilt forward instead of being neatly tucked under as nature intended. An entire realignment of the spine is necessary if posture is to be truly changed.

If you suspect that your posture is contributing to your visual deficiency, look into forms of exercise and therapy that can effect lasting changes. Yoga is excellent and so are all the available forms of bodywork, including the Feldenkrais and Alexander techniques, Bioenergetics exercises, and deep tissue work such as Rolfing and Postural Integration. You'll discover just how good your body can feel as well as experience its influence on your vision.

The kind of *lighting* you spend time under also influences the way you see. Fluorescent lighting can be especially troublesome. To begin with, the level of illumination is so low that there is not enough contrast between dark and light to allow the eyes to function without strain. In the older fluorescent lights, and many are still out there, radiation is emitted as well as a flickering that conflicts with the rate of our body's own vibratory rhythm. This conflict is enormously draining on our stores of vitamins. In addition, these lights do not supply us with the full spectrum of colors available in natural light. These colors are necessary for the proper functioning of our pituitary and pineal glands, which have a profound influence on our health. People who work constantly under fluorescent lights report a high incidence of headaches, colds, and other ailments, including emotional imbalances. A study done some years ago in Florida pointed out just how dramatically these lights can affect us. A class of hyperactive children were separated into two different rooms, one with ordinary fluorescents and the other with special ones that contained the full spectrum of colors. Within a few weeks the children under the full-spectrum lights became noticeably calmer and were able to study more efficiently. Meanwhile, those in the room with the old lights remained hyperactive and unable to concentrate on their studies. If you must work under fluorescent lights, try to convince your employer to install full-spectrum bulbs.

Incandescent lights are not as desirable as sunlight, but they are an improvement on fluorescent bulbs, especially for reading purposes. Whatever light you read under, the old axioms you have heard are true: Hold the print directly in front of you and have the lighting coming over your shoulder. Let me add a special note here about computer *video display terminals* (VDTs), since they are the wave of the future. I had read about the health and vision problems linked to them, but not until I began the process of selecting a computer of my own to speed up the writing of this book did I experience the strain they can cause. In addition to the issue of radiation, many VTDs produce quite a bit of flicker, have very small print, and some lack adequate contrast between the background and the print. Adding to these visual stresses is the placement of the screen. Many are at eye level or higher. The best natural angle for reading is a slightly downward one. Looking straight ahead or up for long periods of time puts enormous strain on the eyes. As I tried out various brands of computers, I found my shoulders and neck tightening and my eyes burning. However, the moment I laid eyes on a laptop model I felt everything relax.

Laptop computers utilize the same liquid crystal display (LCD) of letters that you find in digital clocks. The contrast is quite good in most of them and there is no radiation whatsoever. The screens are generally roomy and the text is displayed at a much lower angle than it is on the more sophisticated permanent models. The choice was obvious for me. I highly recommend these laptops and sincerely hope that the LCD screens will become popular with all computers. If you have to use the TV-type screen, move it off the top of the computer and down to an angle that won't put so much stress on your eyes. As with reading in general, look into the distance as often as possible.

Obviously, your *glasses or contacts* are still an important part of your current visual abilities. Unless your correction is very mild, you're not going to be able to make one swift jump from needing artificial lenses to clear sight. But as your sight improves you are going to have a difficult time utilizing glasses that contain a prescription stronger than you need. Your eyes will automatically attempt to adjust to the lenses, which is a definite step backward. One client of mine did her exercises faithfully but continued to wear her glasses whenever she wasn't actually exercising her eyes. Soon she began to develop severe headaches. They were so intense that she harbored fears of a brain tumor. Fortunately she went to the eye doctor before consulting an expensive neurologist. During the examination the optometrist exclaimed, "This can't be! Your sight has improved. That's not possible!" Improvement, of course, is more than possible, but what was unusual about this case was this woman's eyes maintaining the improvement in spite of the strength of her glasses. This strain had caused the headaches, which vanished as soon as she received a weaker prescription.

If you've been a packrat and saved your old glasses, which are no doubt weaker prescriptions, you can save yourself a lot of money because you can simply work your way back through these lesser corrections. If you don't have old glasses around, you'll most likely need to go to the eye doctor for a weaker set or two before you are free of them altogether or have achieved a satisfactory improvement. In most states a 20/40 correction is acceptable for legal driving. This way your eyes have room to improve. When your sight improves so that you see clearly through this weaker correction, have it reduced again so that there is room for even more improvement. Do be prepared for skepticism and chuckles from your optometrist, but it is completely within your rights to ask for a weaker prescription.

Sunglasses have always been scorned by Bates teachers because they rob the eyes of nutrients and relaxation provided by the sun. Relaxing into healthy sunlight instead of tensing up against it is an easily learned skill. However, I make it a rule of thumb that if the glare is harsh, it is better to wear sunglasses than to tense the eyes. Stay away from the darkest ones, though, as they cause so much dilation in your pupils that dangerous ultraviolet rays can enter your eyes. The vanishing ozone layer and the resultant increase in harmful ultraviolet rays present a real dilemma. However, at this point there is still enough positive value to natural light to allow in what you can comfortably handle. Maintaining our ability to absorb the benefits of sunlight is yet another good reason to become active in the effort to save our environment and atmosphere.

4

What Is Hypnosis?

There are so many misconceptions about hypnosis that even the most trusted sources define it incorrectly—the dictionary, for example. I looked in my handy paperback edition and found: "A sleeplike condition in a person who is then very susceptible to suggestions and acts only if told to do so." Shaking my head over this, I went on to consult the two-thousand-page monster I haul out only for emergencies. It told me: "A sleeplike condition psychically induced, usually by another person, in which the subject loses consciousness but responds, with certain limitations, to the suggestions of the hypnotist." Loses consciousness? Psychically induced? No wonder I have to spend twenty or thirty minutes explaining to new clients just what hypnosis is and isn't before we can get down to work!

I define hypnosis as an intently focused, altered state of consciousness through which one can influence perception, physiological functioning, emotions, and behavior patterns. An altered state of consciousness is completely different from a loss of consciousness. It is also a perfectly natural state of mind. We alter our consciousness all the time. Joy, anger, fear, sorrow, love, and so on—these are all altered states of consciousness. So is the state of mind of the ninety-pound woman who lifts a car off her child. And that of the engrossed reader aware of nothing but her book even though she is in the middle of Grand Central Station. Or of the daydreaming driver who suddenly sees his off ramp but has no idea how he managed to control the car for the last twenty miles. These last three examples of altered states of consciousness are extremely similar to hypnosis, and some would insist that they are self-induced hypnotic states. The only real difference is that what we call hypnosis utilizes conscious suggestions to shift the focus of awareness rather than the shift occurring spontaneously.

Meditation, prayer, Sufi dancing, chanting, autogenic training, progressive relaxation, creative visualization, and Silva Mind Control are examples of consciousness-altering techniques that are also closely related to hypnosis, and, again, some would insist that they are all forms of hypnosis. They all get you into the same part of your brain, the subconscious, but the process known as hypnosis generally involves a specific mental ritual for entering the altered state, followed by goal-oriented instructions. Even though self-hypnosis is an easy procedure, hypnosis is the form of mental discipline that is thought to need most the guidance of another person. One of the great misconceptions about hypnosis is that this guidance is *controlled* by another person.

The reason for this misconception lies in the historical roots of hypnosis. In every known early society there were individuals believed to have the power to cure others' ailments. The healer in primitive cultures utilized rhythm of some sort, be it chanting or drumming or shaking rattles, to induce altered consciousness in the subject, while in more sophisticated societies such as the Egyptian and Greek, priests tended to their patients in "sleep temples." Regardless of what the healer said or did, there was always the belief that he or she was controlling the healing process. We know now that it was the patient's mind that created the healing, but it took thousands of years of social and scientific evolution to recognize this basic fact.

Perhaps the greatest discovery of modern medicine is the placebo effect, which is something the medical profession keeps trying to rule out with double-blind studies. We've all heard the stories about doctors who ran out of anesthetic during wartime. The wounded soldier in terrible pain is given a sugar pill but is told it is morphine. And the pain goes away. The soldier's belief in what morphine would do for him altered his body chemistry, which released endorphins, natural painkillers, from his brain. The relief is real, not imaginary. Recently such enlightened doctors as Bernie Siegel and Carl Simonton have brought mind power, belief, and emotion back into medicine. The era of pure science is coming to an end as we realize that the human factor is at the core of healing.

Drs. Siegel and Simonton and the others who emulate them have their fair share of critics who want all truth to be visible under a microscope, but the tide is turning. For two centuries their forerunners were not only scorned but actually driven out of the medical profession. The most famous of these persecuted souls was the man credited with being the father of hypnosis as we know it. The term used was not hypnosis but mesmerism.

Franz Anton Mesmer was an eighteenth-century Austrian physician who developed a theory known as animal magnetism. He and other doctors believed that healing would occur when the body's magnetic field was properly aligned with that of the earth and the planets. When his patients recovered from their ailments after he passed magnets over their bodies, nobody, including Mesmer, had any idea that it was the suggestions for healing that were producing the physiological changes. The astounding degree of his success aroused jealousy and animosity among his peers, who were founders of the Age of Reason, which demanded that medical findings be substantiated under a microscope. In France, where his treatments were especially popular, the French Academy of Science appointed a committee, which included our own Benjamin Franklin, to investigate Mesmer's findings. The committee concluded that there was no such thing as animal magnetism and that the curative results were due solely to the patients' overactive imaginations. Mesmer was discredited, died in obscurity, and the search for external healing forces continued.

But you can't keep a good idea down. By the 1840s a few curious and sometimes desperate doctors began to reexamine Mesmer's findings. The doctors who gave those sugar pills to the wounded during wars in this century were inspired to do so by a British physician working in a prison hospital in India in the 1840s. Dr. James Esdaile had run out of anesthesia to use before and after surgery, and he was also experiencing the 50 percent postoperative mortality rate that was common at the time. He had heard of mesmeric passes, even without magnets, inducing sleep and anesthesia in patients. He made repetitive hand passes over the suffering men until they lapsed into what is now known as a hypnotic trance. Interestingly, he gave no suggestions. Perhaps the idea of animal magnetism should be looked into further! Not only did Esdaile's patients feel no pain but the mortality rate dropped to 5 percent. When he returned to England his medical license was revoked because of this unorthodox practice. The medical board also judged the low mortality rate to be blasphemous, as it was obvious that God meant men to suffer.

The atmosphere became more tolerant shortly thereafter, and the actual persecution of doctors using the technique ceased. In the 1840s a Scottish physician, James Braid, discovered that mesmeric passes were not necessary to induce this state of mind that looked so much like sleep. He developed the concept of eye fixation and also realized that it was suggestion that triggered the healing response. And it was Braid who named the phenomenon hypnosis, from the Greek word for sleep. As soon as he realized that what was happening wasn't sleep at all, he tried to change the name to "monoideaism," which he defined as "essentially a state of mental concentration, in which the faculties of the mind of the patient are so engrossed with a single idea or train of thought as, for the nonce, to be dead or indifferent to all other considerations and influences." This is an excellent description of what really goes on, but monoideaism is hardly a catchy term. Hypnosis is, and the name stuck.

At this point the new field of psychiatry was beginning to unfold. Doctors quickly learned that hypnosis could cure the mind as well as the body. Some authorities, in fact, credit Mesmer with being the father of psychiatry as well as hypnosis. When the famous Nancy Clinic in France opened in the 1840s, hypnosis was the sole method of treatment. Among the many doctors who went there to study was a young Austrian named Sigmund Freud. He was so impressed that when he returned to Austria he worked alongside the best medical hypnotist he could find. But not for long. The fact was that Freud was a terrible hypnotist. He was authoritarian in manner and disliked making eye contact with his patients. He blamed his failure on hypnosis, took up a seat behind his patients, and so began the technique known as Freudian analysis. It is interesting to note that while Freud's theories of repressed sexuality, free association, and dream analysis took time to catch on in Europe, hypnosis has always been a popular form of therapy there.

Freudian theories were more successful in the United States, while hypnosis languished in obscurity until the world wars. It provided a fast and effective therapy for shell shock and battle fatigue, and of course there were those doctors using suggestion along with sugar pills to alleviate suffering. In 1955 the British Medical Association endorsed it as a valid medical treatment. The American Medical Association followed suit a few years later. The original endorsement was for physiological uses, such as pain relief and postoperative healing, but the psychiatric community joined the bandwagon after the pioneering work of Dr. Milton Erickson. Ericksonian hypnotherapy techniques are studied and utilized by mental health professionals from all schools of thought. The tide has indeed turned. To this day in my own practice I have yet to have a client whose doctor or psychologist has discouraged them from also working with me.

Hypnosis works so well because it bypasses the conscious mind, which is analytical and critical. Hypnosis speaks directly to the master control tower within us, the subconscious mind. This portion of our brain is the seat of our emotions, our beliefs, our habits, and our physiological functioning. All of these basic components are set within the subconscious mind when we are young and impressionable. They can be changed only through extraordinary means or long-term repetition—unless we access the subconscious directly. And that is what hypnosis does. Once we are inside this part of the brain, it is as impressionable as it was when we were young. In essence, we reprogram the subconscious with a new set of operating instructions. It then controls our behavior, both physically and emotionally, with this new information.

The process used for accessing the subconscious through hypnosis is both simple and pleasurable. We don't fully understand why it works the way it does, but the act of imagining physiological sensations alters brain-wave patterns so that the conscious mind is set aside and the subconscious is brought to the forefront. Hypnotic inductions instruct the subject to become actively involved in allowing certain sensations and actions to feel real, even though we all know that it's just a fantasy. These include feeling a downward sensation, a relaxation of muscles, and eyelids so heavy and lazy that they can't be opened. The dictionary's definition of the hypnotic state as being able to act only when told to do so is totally false. The subjects know perfectly well that they could get up or open their eyes if they really wanted to. But it is enjoyable to allow the experience to seem real. I am very careful to explain to new clients that this is not a contest. I am neither going to control them nor am I going to do anything to them. This is a cooperative effort to get them into their deeper mind, and I am simply the guide.

All hypnosis is self-hypnosis. Barring vicious brainwashing techniques, nobody gets into this state of mind who doesn't want to. And there is no place somewhere "out there" that you go to, much less a place you are not able to get back from. It's a journey inside yourself. It feels like coming home to the most peaceful and sane place imaginable.

On this particular journey your destination will be the optic portion of your subconscious. You'll be restructuring this control center of your vision, and it, in turn, will send out signals for the healing and proper functioning of your eyes. The addition of hypnosis to the classic Bates method renders the ensuing vision improvement more effective and permanent than with other techniques. In the past it was very frustrating for me to observe people's sight improve dramatically during a lesson and then revert right back to their old way of seeing once we were finished. The way we see is as ingrained a habit as there can be. We reinforce it every moment we have our eyes open. It takes a powerful force to restructure a habit this entrenched. That force is the subconscious mind, and the tool it uses best is hypnosis.

5

How to Hypnotize Yourself

Even if you are already a skilled hypnotic subject or a hypnotist, be sure to read this chapter carefully. Much of what you will learn here will be used throughout the HypnoVision program. If you are new to hypnosis, take your time in learning the procedure. The success of the program depends on your ability to enter readily and deeply into the hypnotic experience. If you are going to work with a partner, read Chapter 11 before you begin working with the material in this one. Sharing the HypnoVision process with another person can enhance the experience both visually and emotionally. Consider the possibility.

In theory, working under the guidance of a hypnotist, even one trained simply with the material in this chapter, is more effective than going it on your own. This is because we have been so conditioned to accept instructions from authority figures we trust. First our parents, then our teachers and spiritual leaders, then our bosses and doctors, and even, occasionally, our politicians. In addition, you've been following your own directions for how to see for years, and obviously it hasn't gone well; otherwise, you wouldn't be reading this book. You are seeking outside guidance to help restructure your visual functioning, so it makes sense to your subconscious to hear another voice giving these instructions. Also, with this other voice guiding you it's easier to relax to the depths necessary to open up your subconscious. For all these reasons, working in partnership with another person is the ideal scenario. If you can find a partner, even one for part of your program, perhaps the evening sessions, wonderful!

The next-best scenario is to have a person with a good speaking voice record the scripts laid out in the program for you. Take into account whether you feel more comfortable with a male or female voice. You also want to determine if you respond better to an authoritarian tone of voice or one that is more gently persuasive. If even this is not possible, and you will be working alone, you will need to tape-record all the full-length sessions. You will be able to remember the suggestions to give yourself during the backup minisessions, but the long ones are too complicated to commit to memory. You can tape all the sessions at once, but I recommend recording at the beginning of each week so that your voice doesn't end up sounding tired. If you're not wild about the sound of your voice, you'll find that you will get used to it and that it will improve with practice. It will help to insert the following sentence in your first session: "I like and trust the sound of my own voice, and respond positively to all suggestions that I give myself."

Every hypnosis session has four parts. First there is the induction, which consists of the directions you follow to imagine physiological sensations as real. This alters your brain waves and puts you in a hypnotic state. Next comes the deepening process, which, as the name implies, takes you deeper into the trance state. It consists simply of one or more added inductions that again ask you to imagine physical responses as real. Then there are the suggestions themselves. Suggestions are synonymous with directions, but the former term is most commonly used, to remind you that you are the one really in control and that you have the power to accept or reject any suggestion made. Finally there is the awakening procedure. If an emergency should occur during your session, such as the house catching on fire, you would automatically pop out of the hypnotic state and be able to take care of the situation. In fact, any time you want the session to end, you can simply open your eyes while affirming how alert you are. But hypnosis feels so good that most of us really would prefer to remain in that lovely relaxed state of mind. The awakening process reminds your conscious mind that it's time to go back to work now. When you do open your eyes, you'll feel wonderfully refreshed.

What does it feel like to be hypnotized? How do you know if you've really been hypnotized? The biggest misconception about hypnosis, which I have to explain over and over to new clients, is that it doesn't feel "weird." And even at that I still hear many people say after their first session, "Well, I don't know if I was hypnotized. But I do feel more relaxed than I've ever been in my life." Basically, that's it—you simply feel relaxed. It is a natural expectation, of course, that something that can have such an enormous impact on your behavior and well-being would feel unusual, but it doesn't. There are, however, some telltale signs that commonly occur when entering into the hypnotic state. Many people feel a pleasant lazy heaviness, a few feel so light they wonder if they are floating, and there is occasionally some falling asleep in the arms and legs as the circulation concentrates in the brain. Some of us experience a particular sensation the moment our brain-wave pattern changes. I always feel a pleasant sinking sensation inside my head that is accompanied by a sigh and a release in my neck muscles, which brings my head down toward my chest if I'm not lying down. An increase in swallowing, fluttering of the eyelids, and occasional twitches in the hands or feet are other signs of hypnosis that occur often. And once in a while someone is lucky enough or becomes skilled enough to become what we call a somnambulist. This tiny fraction of subjects enter so deeply into the hypnotic state that their conscious mind drifts off completely. The first time this happens they generally think they have fallen asleep. But they know the truth when they find their emotions and behavior altered for the better.

Most of us are not fortunate enough to turn our conscious mind off entirely. It tries to maintain its control by becoming what I refer to as "the babbler." One moment you're enjoying following suggestions for heavy eyelids, or whatever, and the next you are suddenly remembering that you have to pick up milk at the store on the way home. This is the most common form of resistance to hypnosis. The trick is not to get caught up in it. Just chuckle at the thought, boot it out of your awareness, and bring yourself back to concentrating on the directions being given. It doesn't matter if you have to do this a hundred times, just don't get involved in dwelling on it. Occasional stray thoughts are to be expected, and they won't negatively impact your hypnotic experience so long as you keep sending them away. The other most common form of resistance is an itch, most often on the nose. Go ahead and scratch it! That won't bring you out of hypnosis, but fixating on an unscratchable itch will. So, scratch, change your position, or whatever, just don't lie or sit there and worry about how you're doing it wrong and it's not working for you. There is no real right or wrong way to be hypnotized, there's only your experience. Relax and enjoy it. If you are a hyperope with the characteristic outward nature, you may find yourself a little challenged by resistance to the inward nature of hypnosis. Just stick with it; it's worth the effort!

Your main job is to activate your wonderful childlike imagination and play along with the idea of the suggestions feeling like reality. The specific sensations you will be exploring are your muscles expanding and then relaxing, a downward movement, and your eyelids being so heavy and relaxed that they refuse to budge when you attempt to open them. It's just a little game of imagination, but it will open the door to your subconscious.

The HypnoVision program set out in this book, which takes four to eight weeks depending on your visual dysfunction, consists of two full-length sessions (about twenty to thirty minutes each) and an average of three minisessions (about three to five minutes each) a day. If this absolutely won't fit into your schedule, do what you can and allow the process to take longer. For the full ones there are lengthy inductions, deepening, and suggestions. For the minis you'll be using what is called a rapid induction, followed by brief deepening and suggestions. Although I encourage the use of the long induction for the full sessions, you may use the rapid induction if you truly feel you enter a deep state of hypnosis with it. When you move on to the program itself, the only differences will be that the suggestions will change and you will be adding a technique that Dr. Bates developed, known as palming. By cupping your palms over your closed eyes, you give them the added relaxation of the darkness and the warmth, and it appears that electromagnetic energy flows through our palms and aids in the healing process.

The inductions, deepenings, and awakenings that you will learn in this chapter are exactly the same as those you will use later in the HypnoVision program. The suggestions will be shorter—just enough to give you a positive attitude about what you are about to undertake and to experience the standard benefits of hypnosis, such as relaxation and self-confidence.

If you are going to tape the induction and deepening directions that follow, or have someone else tape them for you, now is the time to do it. Be sure to read at a leisurely pace, with plenty of pauses. I've used ellipses to indicate the places needing the longest pauses. Don't skip over anything that seems repetitive; it is all there for an important purpose.

Now all you need is a comfortable place to sit or lie down—a recliner chair is ideal. Unhook your phones and make sure you won't be disturbed. Once the tape machine is on, or a friend is ready to read, get comfortable and close your eyes. Let that creative imagination flow and become involved in the following:

o

". . . Allow yourself to begin to relax. . . . Focus your attention on your breathing. As you feel the gentle rising and falling of your chest, let your breathing expand just a little. Feel your chest rise with each breath in and fall with each breath out. Slow down the whole process just a little. . . . As you breathe be aware that there are three parts to each breath. There's that gentle expansion, then that pleasant sense of letting go as you exhale, and then there's a peaceful moment of stillness before you spontaneously draw air in again as you need it. Be aware of that peaceful pause. . . . Be aware that there's a pleasant, almost massagelike, sensation to your breathing. The gentle stretching as you breathe in, the letting go as you breathe out, and that peaceful pause before you next breathe in. . . . That feeling of letting go as you breathe out is exactly what relaxation feels like. Focus on it fully, for in a few moments that is what you will begin to feel throughout your body. . . . Begin to activate your creative imagination now. Pretend that you're like a balloon and that you can blow up any part of yourself that you wish. You'll be feeling this sensation of being like a balloon, but if you get a visual image as well, that's fine. What color would you be if you were a balloon? . . . Let your whole torso, but not your arms, legs, or head, be like a balloon now. As you inhale spread that feeling of expansion to include everything from the top of your shoulders to the bottom of your hips. Expanding as you breathe in, going limp and loose as you breathe out, just like a balloon with the air going out of it. Expanding, relaxing, and also enjoying the peaceful pause in between. . . . All the muscles and organs in your torso melting into relaxation with each easy breath out. . . . It feels good to let go and relax. . . . Now let each breath in feel as if it is flowing down inside your arms to the tips of your fingers as well as throughout your torso.

"Your arms, hands, and torso rising as you inhale, falling as you exhale. . . . Melting into deeper and more lazy relaxation with each easy breath out. . . . Now expand that feeling of breathing into yourself down into your legs as well. Feel your breath seem to flow down through your torso and into your legs and feet to the tips of your toes. Feel expansion as you breathe in and a complete letting go, almost sinking down into the surface beneath you, with each breath out. . . . Melting deeper into lazy comfort with each easy breath out. . . . Lazy, loose, and limp. . . . This letting go will continue with each breath out as you now bring your attention to your neck and throat and realize you can let go there as well. You may find yourself swallowing as your throat relaxes. . . . Be aware of the hinges of your jaws and allow them to loosen. You may notice your teeth unclenching as you relax your jaw. And let that loosening sweep down your face in a wave of letting go. Around your mouth, into your lips, even your tongue is a muscle that can let go and relax. . . . Be aware of your eyelids and let them spread out more over your eyes. Feel your eyes relaxing as well. Letting go. Let your eyebrows soften and that space between them seem to widen. As relaxation moves up into your forehead, you can feel it smooth out. As the relaxation moves into your scalp, you may experience a tingling sensation as it flows over your head. Over the top, down the back and around your ears, and then down into your neck. Down into your shoulders and upper back. Softening. . . . Letting go from the top of your head to the tips of your toes with each easy breath out. . . . Drifting into deeper and more comfortable relaxation with each breath out. . . . In a few moments now you'll be able to take that relaxation even deeper while I count down from ten to one.

"Every time you hear a number, let yourself experience a downward sensation, just as if you were in an elevator starting down to the next floor. By the number one you may find yourself more pleasantly, deeply relaxed than ever before. Imagine moving down now—Ten. Drifting gently downward. Nine—every muscle letting go as you move down. Eight—every muscle, nerve, and cell relaxing. Seven—down into deeper and deeper relaxation. Six—so comfortably, wonderfully relaxed. Five—halfway down now, feeling lazy and comfortable. Four—even your eyes let go as you sink ever downward. Three—deeper and deeper down. Two—lazy and comfortable. And yet you can double your present relaxation when you hear the next number. You may feel this as a deep sinking sensation or as a wave of letting go from the top of your head to the tips of your toes. Moving down to number one, doubling your relaxation. . . . So wonderfully, deeply relaxed. Your mind, your body, and your entire visual system in a state of total peace and relaxation. . . . But you can take this relaxation even deeper. Bring your attention to your eyelids. What would it feel like if they were even more relaxed, loose, and heavy? So loose and heavy that even as you try to open them they won't budge. All you feel is a slight fluttering in your lids, and that sends waves of relaxation through you. Let go of that unsuccessful effort, and feel

yourself sink even deeper into pleasant, lazy relaxation. . . . Luxuriate in these sensations of relaxation and well-being.⊖*
. . . Relaxing this deeply has a regenerating effect on both your mind and your body. Every function, every system, organ, and muscle within you benefits from this total relaxation. Your mind and your body are coming into balance and harmony with each other. You feel a deep sense of well-being and inner peace. You are filled with self-confidence and realize that you are capable of fulfilling all your potentials. It is your birthright to develop your potentials and become all you were meant to be. Clear, relaxed vision is one of these potentials, and you are confident of achieving it. You deserve the best in life, including clear vision, and you feel good about your decision to make positive changes. When you return to full waking consciousness, you will feel refreshed, confident, and positive about your future. . . . In a few moments I'm going to begin counting from one to five. These numbers will serve two very different purposes. At the subconscious level you will more fully accept and integrate every positive suggestion that I've made. At the conscious level these numbers will serve as signals to your conscious mind that it is time to return to full waking consciousness. By the number five you'll be wide awake and refreshed, as if you've just had the best night's sleep of your life. . . . One—starting to come up now. Let your breaths begin to deepen as you draw in energy. Two—coming up, breaths expanding. Feeling rested. Three—halfway up now, aware that even your eyes feel refreshed. They feel cool and moist. Four—almost all the way back. Aware of the clothes on your body and the surface beneath you. Ready to come all the way back when you hear the next number. All the way now—five. Take in a deep breath, you may also want to stretch, and when you open your eyes you'll be fully alert, feeling terrific, infused with calm energy and a deep inner sense of well-being."

o

* The function of the symbol will be explained on page 55.

Again, let me encourage you not to rush through your practice with this initial session. Use it to fully develop your skill as a hypnotic subject and, of course, your speaking voice and tone if you are not working with a partner. You don't want to waste any of your actual HypnoVision sessions on still being in the learning process. Once you feel you are an accomplished hypnotic subject, move on to learning the rapid induction technique that follows.

With a little practice you can induce self-hypnosis in a matter of seconds. Once you respond readily to the procedure you've just learned, you'll be able to modify it for a rapid induction. You may even soon discover that you don't need all three steps of rapid induction. But shorten it further only if and when you are sure you can enter the hypnotic state that quickly. You won't need to tape the procedure; it's short and simple enough to memorize. You also don't need to say anything out loud; just think the suggestions.

For the first stage you'll use a combination of visualization, numbers, and your breath to quickly induce that pleasant and by-now-familiar sensation of letting go from head to toe as you exhale. As soon as you close your eyes, take a moment to state to yourself mentally but very clearly that you are about to enter rapidly into a deep state of hypnosis. Then count the number one to yourself as you take a deep breath in, feel yourself expand, and visualize yourself as a *green* balloon blowing up. Then, as you let the breath out and feel your muscles let go, imagine your green balloon-self with the air going out, becoming completely limp, while you mentally affirm "relaxed." Then comes the next breath, the expansion and the mental count of two accompanied by the image of a *blue* balloon-self. As you let the breath out, feel the letting go and see the blue balloon deflating and going limp, you say to yourself "more relaxed." Then, counting three to yourself, inhale once more, this time seeing a *purple* balloon-self inflating. As you let the breath out, feel the letting go and see the purple balloon with all the air going out of it, and affirm "completely relaxed."

Next you mentally count down from three to one, feeling that downward sensation taking you deeper with each number down. Finally you bring your attention to your eyelids, let them loosen even more, tell yourself they won't open no matter how hard you try, and then try unsuccessfully to open them. Give up the effort and feel yourself to be lazy, comfortable, and hypnotized.

For your practice runs, try giving yourself abbreviated versions of the suggestions included in the previous practice session. Just remember the gist of them and mentally phrase them in a way that sounds good to you. Then remind yourself that the count from one up to three will bring you into fully conscious alertness. Count up one number at a time, each time mentally affirming that you are becoming alert, awake, and refreshed. Open your eyes after the number three, and you will indeed be alert and refreshed and just have given yourself a wonderful hypnosis minisession. Even when you are no longer doing your vision improvement work, you'll find that adding both the complete and minisessions to your life on a regular basis will greatly enhance the quality of your life.

There is one more procedure to learn before you begin the program in earnest. This is the use of the pendulum, technically known as the Chevreul pendulum. Chevreul was a nineteenth-century French chemist and the first person to understand that the subconscious mind can communicate through what we refer to as ideomotor responses. These are tiny muscular reflexes in our fingers that reflect subconscious answers to "yes" and "no" questions. These reflex movements control the directional swing of the pendulum. There is no hocus-pocus here. The technique has withstood the test of time and has long been utilized by the most eminent of medical and psychiatric hypnotherapists, such as Drs. Milton Erickson, David Cheek, and Ernest Rossi. It has a wide range of applications, from the uncovering of psychological causes behind physical and mental dysfunctions to mundane uses, such as discovering where you left your car keys. You will be using it during the HypnoVision program to reveal what additional work you need to do if you haven't achieved your desired degree of improvement in the allotted time. Your subconscious knows what needs to be done and will tell you through the pendulum.

All you need is a piece of string and a paper clip, although you may use something more exotic, such as a ring or a crystal if you like. Your string should be about a foot long. Tie your paper clip or other shiny object securely and make sure it is evenly balanced. Rest your elbow on a table and let the string dangle. Let it come to a standstill. Now you'll establish yes, no, I-don't-know, and I'm-not-ready-to-talk-about-it answers.

First, think "yes." Be aware of the affirmative quality of the word. You may even want to close your eyes and visualize a green neon sign continually flashing "yes." There is a finely tuned neuromotor connection between your brain and your fingertips. Before long the pendulum will begin to swing in a particular direction, either front and back, right to left, a diagonal or a circular motion. Give it time to be fully established and note the direction of the swing.

Now begin thinking "no." How does a negative response feel emotionally? See a red neon sign flashing "no" if you like. Soon the pendulum will slow to a stop and then change the direction of its swing. This is your "no" answer.

Go through the same procedure for "I don't know" and "I'm not ready to talk about it." Concentrate on the emotional feelings involved in each of these responses. The I'm-not-ready-to-talk-about-it response may occur later if you ask if there are emotional reasons why you don't yet see clearly. If that happens, it's time to do some deep personal examination and perhaps seek out professional help. It is more likely, however, that you will simply find out you need more work on a particular exercise.

Each time you use the pendulum, it is necessary to reestablish your directional answers. We don't know why, but sometimes the responses in our motor system differ from time to time. (By the way, this handy method can also be a useful addition to your daily life.)

Now it's time to really get down to work. You're already involved in the adventure, and it's just going to get better from here on in.

6

The Myopia Program

Ahead of you, fellow myope, is a wondrous journey from near-sighted to clearsighted. Some of you may simply experience changes in your eyesight, but the majority of you will also experience an expansion of your personality as well. No endeavor I've ever engaged in has changed me so deeply and in so many ways as did working with my vision. "Vision" is certainly the appropriate term here, as opposed to eyesight, because the vast majority of myopes display a nearsightedness in their personalities as well as in their eyes. I have yet to work with a single myope who did not have an emotional as well as a visual coming-out during the process of changing his or her eyesight.

Consider yourself, and see if some of the following descriptions apply to you. Are you more of an introvert than an extrovert? Are you a verbalizer rather than a visualizer? Do you read a lot? Do you pay closer attention to details rather than the big picture? Do you tend to engage in intellectual or artistic pursuits rather than sports? Are you more of a loner than a joiner? Do you tend to examine and analyze events and emotions rather than feel and respond to them? Do you need the approval of others to confirm your own beliefs? Do you walk away from confrontations rather than take action? Do you carry a lot of tension in your shoulders, neck, and jaw? Are you more tall than short and slender as opposed to heavy? Were there people and events in your early years that were emotionally if not downright physically threatening, such as divorce or abuse in the family or overly strict parents, teachers, or religious figures?

In every workshop I give there are always a few myopes who don't fit the mold, but most of us do. Basically, there are personality factors and emotional responses within us that create a visual field that is drawn in to a close, safe distance. Even when we outgrow or compensate for these tendencies, the visual habits and muscular tensions remain. During the process of bringing your vision up to match your personal growth, you may very well discover that you also clear up any lingering vestiges of your old behavior patterns as well. As you free your vision, you'll free your whole being at the same time.

If you are a musician, you will have both added opportunity and challenge through this program. It appears that many musicians subconsciously suppress their visual sense in order to enhance their innate musical ability. Mesmer became aware of this in early work when he cured a blind young woman who was also a musical prodigy on the piano. When she regained her sight and, interestingly, her sense of smell, she lost much of her musical ability. Fortunately, this doesn't have to be the case, and, in fact, musical talent can actually be enhanced while restoring clarity of vision. I have seen this marvelous development occur in several musicians I have worked with. The key is to add suggestions for the visual expansion to bring about a corresponding expansion in the musical sense. They can indeed go hand in hand, it's just a matter of making this clear to the subconscious. Those of us who aren't musicians won't develop musical talent through vision improvement, but we'll expand in other realms.

Hypnosis, by the way, can greatly enhance existing musical ability without vision being a part of the equation. Rachmaninoff, for example, sought help from a hypnotist because of a paralyzing musical block, and the treatment was so successful that he went on to create the masterpieces he is now known for. One in particular, "Rhapsody on a Theme of Paganini," is one of the most beautiful pieces ever composed. You may know it as the central theme to the movie *Somewhere in Time*. This magnificent music was what my husband and I chose to have played at our wedding. I didn't find out about Rachmaninoff's experience with hypnosis until sometime later, but it made the piece even more meaningful for me.

During the eight-week program laid out here, you'll be progressively building your attitudes and belief system about your sight, your visual skills and habits, and the ability of your brain to direct physiological changes and healing in the structure of your eyes. Each phase builds on the one before it and readies you for the one that follows. The ideal program is set out here, consisting of two full sessions of twenty to thirty minutes each and three or more minisessions of three to five minutes each. The full sessions are designed so that one is done in the morning and the other in the evening. If you can't meet this schedule, don't give up. Do what you can when you can and allow for the whole program to take longer than eight weeks. On the other hand, it is possible that you will progress faster than the prepared schedule. There's no exact formula that suits us all. We're all different, and it is up to each of us to develop our own perception of how to bring about changes within. Look within, be flexible, and, above all, be kind and gentle to yourself as you undertake this adventure.

Each session begins with an induction you learned in Chapter 5, either the rapid or the full-length one. In the interest of time, you will probably lean toward the rapid induction. This is fine so long as you really feel those sensations of letting go, moving downward, and eyelids unable to open that tell you you're hypnotized. If you use your taped full-length induction, start your new taped suggestions where you see the symbol (the ◕) on page 49. Each week you can tape over the suggestions for the previous week, or you can create a whole new tape for each week. If you find you have more work to do before achieving your goal, you may need the session later on. If you are using the rapid induction, you will, of course, simply go over it in your mind and then go on to your tape of the suggestions for the session. Awakening procedures are supplied along with the suggestion scripts, as they contain specific reinforcements of the subject of each session.

Don't skip over what may appear to be a lot of repetitive words or phrases. They are there for a purpose. Repetition is one way to achieve change at the subconscious level. The combination of repetition and hypnosis is an ideal situation. There's a lot of negative programming to be overcome, and we'll be using every technique possible to change the "program" to a positive one.

During the next eight weeks you can expect to experience a wide variety of visual and emotional highs, lows, and plateaus. Change rarely occurs evenly and consistently. The learning of new skills tends to be erratic, and the old habits put up a fight to maintain their dominance. Being able to share and discuss your thoughts, progress, and moments of insecurity is another good reason to work with a partner if you can find a compatible one. For example, Charles and Diana, who, of course, never got over chuckling about their names, were partners I set up together because they had similar degrees of myopia. They also discovered that they shared similar childhood experiences at an especially strict Catholic school. Their tears and laughter over the discipline handed out by dark-robed figures wielding paddles and the fears that nearly anything they did might send them to Hell were valuable aids to their emotional and visual healing.

Another helpful means of reflection is keeping what I call an Eyelogue, a daily diary of your journey into clear vision. Review it often as you go along and you will be buoyed up by the evidence of your ever-growing visual awareness and clarity. I had to do most of my visual retraining on my own, so my only sounding board was the diary I kept. I dubbed it my Eyelogue, and this account of my experiences eventually formed the basis for my first book, *Visionetics.* An Eyelogue is especially supportive as you learn to function without your glasses.

From now on go without your glasses whenever you can function comfortably. The general rule of thumb is the same as with sunglasses—use them only when going without would cause strain. As soon as possible obtain a pair of glasses with the prescription reduced to 20/40 so that your eyes will have that all-important room to improve. However, don't discard the stronger pair yet, as you may need them for safe and comfortable night driving (night vision is slow to improve). Remember, there's no law that says you have to see 20/20 all the time. Even more important is that using a weaker prescription will in no way damage your vision. Neither will going without glasses completely, unless one eye is dramatically weaker than the other, in which case depth perception could be impaired since the brain simply ignores inputs from the weak eye.

Beginning with your very first session, your visual system will begin to function better. In the past, you subconsciously tensed up and tried to force clearer vision. Now your subconscious will learn that it is relaxation that will bring about clarity. The blur will gradually clear as you look around you with your newly acquired visual skills. In the meantime, allow yourself into this blur, examining what you see for what it is rather than what it is not. And, of course, always do your sessions without your glasses.

WEEK ONE

As you progress you will be incorporating exercises and massages into your sessions, but this first week will consist of one straight hypnosis session repeated twice a day and reinforced by frequent minisessions (those start on page 63). Once you have induced a hypnotic state, the suggestions will be for relaxation of your eyes and visual system, a readiness for change, and an absolute conviction that these changes will occur. It was not until I became a hypnotherapist that I realized how much a deeply ingrained negative belief system could hold back visual progress. Many people worked diligently but still didn't really believe that they were capable of significant change. You will now be starting your program with this all-important basic restructuring of belief in yourself and your healing abilities. With this groundwork done, you'll find you progress rapidly once the real work begins. Don't skimp on these sessions. Your subconscious needs this vital information.

Whereas you may have reclined for the initial training sessions, you may find that you prefer to sit in front of a table from now on. You will be palming your eyes while you are hypnotized, and you might prefer to do this with the support of a table under your

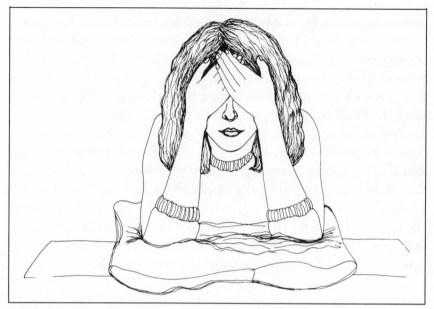

Palming

elbows. However, if you prefer the reclining position, you can give
your arms suggestions for lightness and comfort, and you can even
place pillows under them for support. Play with various possibilities
and pick the one you are the most comfortable with.

Palming, as I mentioned earlier, consists simply of covering your
closed eyes with cupped palms. Don't actually press your palms
against your lids. You're trying to achieve an environment of soothing dark warmth in which your eyes seem to float in relaxation. If
you press the top part of your palm over the bony ridge under your
eyebrows and the bottom of your palm on the bones under your
eyes, you'll create a pleasant vacuum in which your eyes can feel
suspended. You can palm during the induction if you like, but I've
found that many people relax more deeply if they enter the hypnotic state with their arms and hands as relaxed as the rest of their
bodies, and then begin palming along with the suggestions. For that
reason, although I have written the suggestion section that follows
to begin with palming, you may make an adjustment in the script if
you prefer a different order.

Before you begin, go back and take a good look at the illustrations of the normal, myopic, and hyperopic eyes on page 23. Many of your suggestions and visualizations will center on the physical changes that must take place in your eyes, so you need to know the optimal shape. The ability to visualize is not always easy for myopes initially, but it is a skill you will learn. Just today, before sitting down to my writing, I read of yet another study that verifies that the ability to visualize aids in physiological healing. Don't try to force this skill. Just relax and "think" about what is being described and soon your eye/brain will get the hang of it.

Now you're ready to go. Create that quiet time and space twice a day, preferably morning and evening, and begin your hypnotic experience with the induction from Chapter 5, beginning on page 46. At its conclusion (where the asterisk is), go right on with the following:

o

"Now that you're deeply relaxed, cup your hands over your closed eyes in the palming position. Feel how your eyes immediately relax more deeply as they are surrounded by the comforting darkness. The pressure of your hands above and below your eyes allows them to feel like they are floating in the soothing darkness and warmth. Your eyes enjoy letting go and relaxing. Your shoulders, neck, and arms remain comfortable and relaxed. . . . Healing warmth and energy flow from the palms of your hands into your eyes. Your eyes are letting go more and more with each of your easy breaths out. . . . Your ciliary and oblique extraocular muscles are relaxing more and more. They are relaxing so much that your lenses and eyeballs are free to come into a rounder shape. . . . Your eyes and your entire visual system are ready and willing to make positive changes that will bring you clear vision at all distances. . . . You deserve to see clearly at all distances. You deserve to see clearly in the distance, and your eyes and brain are capable of making the changes that will bring you clear vision. . . . You and your visual system are ready, willing, and able to make positive changes in your vision. You and your visual system are ready, willing, and able to make positive changes in your vision. . . . You enjoy seeing clearly, and you know that soon you will see as clearly in the distance as you do close up. As you absorb this fact, realize that it is one that emotionally pleases you. . . . This sense of pleasure increases the relaxation in your ciliary and extraocular muscles. They are relaxing more and more with each moment you remain in this deeply relaxed state of mind. . . . You are emotionally ready to see the world clearly. You realize that shutting out a clear view of the world was an inappropriate response. Now you are ready to see the world clearly. You are a competent, capable, and intelligent individual, and you have a strong sense of your own personal power. . . . You are completely confident of your ability to heal your vision, and you are ready to see the world clearly. You are completely confident of your ability to heal your vision, and you are ready to see the world clearly. . . . You are on an exciting journey into clearer vision, and you enjoy the whole process of changing your sight for the better. Just the thought of this further relaxes your ciliary and extraocular muscles. . . . There is no healing force on earth more powerful than the human mind, your mind. You have the power and ability to change your sight for the better. You are completely confident that you will see more clearly with each passing day. You feel positive and excited about improving your vision. You know you will soon see clearly at all distances. . . . Your visual system is ready for change, and at this very moment your ciliary and extraocular muscles are relaxing and changing. Your eyes can round out now that they are so wonderfully relaxed. . . . Begin feeling that letting go and relaxation now. Just as you imagined your breath filling your whole body, now imagine that each breath in fills and expands your eyes and the muscles that surround them. Experience a gentle stretching sensation with each breath in, followed by a feeling of letting go with each breath out. . . . Gently expanding and stretching, then letting go into lazy, comfortable relaxation. Letting go a little more with each easy breath out. . . . Notice that this feels like a massage. . . . Gently stretching, completely letting go. Letting go.

Letting go. . . . Now add a visual image to this sensation. Any image that works for you is fine. See as well as feel those ciliary and oblique muscles stretching as you breathe into them and releasing and relaxing as you breathe out. See and feel that pleasant letting go. It feels good, experience it, see it. . . . You are ready for this positive change, and it feels good. . . . A pleasant letting go, a melting into deep relaxation within your eye muscles. . . . As the muscles relax your eyeballs are free to come into a rounder shape. See and feel this happening. . . . It feels so good as the muscles relax and your eyes round out. You are ready for this change and your eye muscles, eyeballs, and entire visual system cooperate. The optic center of your brain will continue to send signals for relaxation and expansion of your eyes and your vision. . . . See and feel the expansion, the rounding, the relaxation. . . . Now let the image and the deep breathing into your eyes go for now. Feel the results of what you have done. Your eyes are wonderfully relaxed and the circulation into them has dramatically increased. Notice that your eyes feel moist as well as relaxed. . . . Positive changes have occurred. The optic center of your brain will now continue to send out relaxation signals to your eyes. You are ready for these positive changes, and your mind and visual system are completely capable of achieving these changes. . . . From now on, when you look into the distance your ciliary and oblique muscles will relax, and you will see more clearly. Not only are you ready for positive visual change but you enjoy the process of developing your vision. This is an exciting and wonderful time in your life. You have the confidence and personal power to achieve the changes you desire. Luxuriate for a few moments in that feeling of confidence and power. . . . You're ready for change, you're completely capable of improving your vision, and you feel wonderful about it. . . . In a few moments I'm going to begin counting from one to five. The counting of these numbers will serve two very different purposes. At the subconscious level they will allow this part of your mind to accept and integrate even more fully every positive sugges-

tion that I have made. On the conscious level they will signal
this part of your mind that it is time to come back to full
waking alertness. With each number up, you will feel more
energized, and when we reach number five you will be fully
alert, feeling terrific. . . . Let's start now. One—deepen your
inhalations and feel yourself coming up. . . . Two—so wonderfully relaxed and so completely confident of your ability
to improve your vision. . . . Three—halfway up now. Feeling
so rested and refreshed. Even your eyes feel refreshed and
moist. . . . Four—almost all the way back now. Feeling energy
flow within you with each breath in. Feeling confident and
positive about your vision. When I count the next number,
bring yourself all the way back. Five—take in a deep breath,
remove your hands from your eyes but keep them closed as
you take a stretch and perhaps a yawn. Feeling wide awake
and completely refreshed. Take your time opening your eyes,
and when you do, blink them softly as you gently swing or roll
your head from side to side while your eyes readjust to the
light. . . . Enjoy your ever-increasing visual relaxation and
clarity."

○

There you have it. After letting these suggestions sink into your
subconscious twice a day for a week, your whole being, eyes, mind,
and emotions will not only be ready for change but you will also
most likely experience a feeling of freedom in your vision. The
more you go without your glasses, the more you will be able to see
the difference. You can't overdo these sessions, and I realize that
most of you won't have the time, but I urge you to indulge yourself
in some extra sessions if you can. Even if this isn't a possibility for
you, be sure to use the minisession (beginning on page 63) three
times in between the full ones.

These minis will serve as reinforcement for the full sessions.
Remember that you've been negatively reinforcing your unclear
vision for years; undoing this takes a lot of subconscious work.
Taking a few minutes now and then to remind your eyes to remain
relaxed will be well worth the effort. In addition, your mind and

body will receive a wonderful regenerating boost from these brief sessions. You'll find your spirits and energy riding high.

Read over the following suggestions until you have the concepts within them committed to memory. The exact wording is not crucial, but the ideas are. After using your rapid induction, repeat the key phrases and concepts over and over to yourself for as much time as you have available. Then count yourself up into full awareness, reaffirming your relaxed eyes and positive energy. Notice that these suggestions are presented in the first person, since you'll simply be talking to yourself. Some people like to tape their minisessions and then take the recorder to work. If this idea appeals to you, remember to record the sessions in the second person—"you" instead of "I"—so there is that feeling of having a hypnotist with you. Here is what to think while you are hypnotized in the minisession:

o

"As I cup my hands over my closed eyes, I feel them relax deeply. With each breath in I feel my eyes gently expand, and with each breath out I feel them relax. My ciliary and oblique muscles relax more deeply with each breath out, and my eyeballs become shorter from front to back. . . . Whenever I look into the distance, these muscles relax even more. . . . My visual system is completely capable of changing so that I see clearly at all distances. I am ready to see clearly. I deserve to see clearly. I am completely confident that my vision is improving with each passing day. I enjoy the process of healing my vision. My eyes are wonderfully relaxed. I can feel that they are moist with circulation, energy, and relaxation. Completely refreshed. My vision is improving. . . ."

o

I have witnessed some very mild cases of myopia clear up almost completely with just these beginning sessions. Most of us take longer, of course, but you will no doubt experience a sense of freedom in your vision this week, if not some actual improvement. Almost without exception these initial sessions also result in delightful feelings of relaxation all through the shoulders, neck, and face as well as the eyes themselves. But that's just the beginning. During the second week of the program you will experience relaxation in these areas, all vital to vision, such as you have never known before.

WEEK TWO

In almost all cases of myopia there is corresponding tension in the shoulders, neck, jaw, and facial muscles. There is a vicious cycle going on here; the visual tension creates the bodily tension and then these tight areas keep the eyes restricted. This cycle must be stopped, so now that we've addressed the tension in your specific eye muscles, we'll move on to relaxing the areas tied in to them. Massage while under hypnosis will be your ticket to feelings of muscular freedom and relaxation.

Massage is healing, there's no doubt about it. I learned early in my vision work just how profoundly it could affect vision. But the effects were often temporary. When I added hypnosis to massage, I discovered immediately that the relaxation was not only more deep but also more permanent. After learning what I call Hypno-Massage, the vast majority of my clients are astounded with the degree of openness they experience in their vision, to say nothing of the delightful sensations of muscular freedom. It's a real coming out, and I'm sure you'll enjoy it immensely.

Each of your full sessions will entail a different massage technique. The first is an overall massage that begins with your upper back and shoulders, moves over your head, and then into your face. Every place you'll be working with is directly connected to your eye muscles and your visual system. Massage alone would affect your vision, but its power will be intensified by direct and specific suggestions. The second session is an acupressure massage that was developed by the Chinese thousands of years ago. While it is relaxing, its major purpose is to open the flow of energy into your eyes and visual system. The constriction in myopic eyes creates a very low energy level. As your energy level rises through the massage, your eyes will regain their vitality and power. The directions and suggestions are simple and repetitive, but taping them is still crucial so that your conscious mind doesn't have any work to do.

You can do the morning massage even before you get out of bed. It's a great way to start your day! Be sure that you are surrounded by peace and quiet so that the hypnosis will be fully effective. And feel free to use any or all of it at any other time of the day or night when the idea occurs to you. It's another good thing you can't overdo.

After your standard induction, your tape will go on with the following:

o

"Keep your eyes closed and sit comfortably with your head hanging forward and down. Stretch your arms up, and then bend them at the elbows so that your hands come to rest on either side of your spine, as far down on your upper back as you can reach. Now dig the fingers of your right hand gently but firmly into the muscle next to your spine. With a strong stroke pull your hand out and up, taking it all the way over your shoulder. Then do the same thing in the opposite direction with your left hand. Keep stroking and massaging, hand over hand, as you very slowly work your way up your spine toward your neck. . . . With each stroke of your hands the muscles in your back and shoulders are warming and relaxing. . . . Warming, relaxing, and letting go. . . . This relaxation flows up your spine, into your visual center, and into your eyes themselves. It's as if you were also massaging your eyes. . . . Your circulation is opening and flowing more freely into your back, shoulders, and eyes. . . . Your muscles enjoy the experience of relaxation, and they will maintain it even after you are through with the massage. . . . You breathe into your muscles as you massage them, and this helps them relax more deeply. . . . Feeling more relaxed with each stroke. . . . When you reach your neck, shorten your strokes and keep on massaging. Pull the skin and muscles out and away from your spinal column. Your neck muscles relax into the massage. . . . Your eye muscles are relaxing along with your neck muscles. Be thorough as you work your way up your neck to the base of your skull. . . . Warming, loosening, relaxing. . . . It feels so good to massage your neck. . . . Your neck enjoys the feeling of relaxation and will maintain it even when you finish massaging. You can feel circulation flowing up into your neck and on into your eyes. . . . It feels so good to massage your neck. . . . Your eyes are relaxing along with your neck. . . . When you reach the base of your skull, change the position of your hands so that they are spread out over the back of your head and your thumbs are together at the point where your neck joins your head. Begin massaging in small circular motions with your thumbs along the bony ridge at the base of your skull. Gradually separate your thumbs as you massage and work your way out to the areas under your ears. . . . A firm circular massaging motion. . . . This relaxes the optic center of your brain. . . . About halfway to your ears you will discover indentations that are tender to the touch. These are acupressure points that affect your vision. Give them extra attention. . . . Relaxation flowing in, circulation opening. . . . This area will remain relaxed and energized even when you are finished massaging. . . . When you reach the areas under your ears, massage your way back to the center. . . . Breathe into the massage and feel it expand. . . . Give those tender spots some more extra attention. . . . Relaxed, energized, circulation flowing openly. . . . After your thumbs come together again, begin massaging your scalp with your fingers. Dig them in a little and shake your scalp loose from your skull. . . . After loosening one area, move your fingers to another. Work your way gradually over every part of your scalp. . . . Muscles relaxing. . . . Circulation opening. . . . The loosening and the circulation flow into your eyes as you massage. . . . Your scalp is alive with relaxed energy, and it will remain so even when you are finished with the massage. . . . Let your breath flow into your scalp as you massage it. . . . When you are finished with your scalp, move your thumbs down to the hinges of your jaws next to the bottom of your ears. Allow your jaws to loosen as you massage. . . . Letting go and relaxing. . . . Deep, comfortable relaxation. Your jaws enjoy being relaxed and will remain so even after you finish massaging them. . . . As the hinges of your jaws relax, so do your eyes. Next spread your fingers over your forehead. Move it up and down, back and forth, and around in circles. . . . Feel it loosen and relax. . . . As it does, so do your eyes. . . . This relaxation in your forehead will help your blinking to be more spontaneous and relaxed. . . . Even when you are finished massaging your forehead, it will remain loose and relaxed. . . . Now grasp your eyebrows between your thumbs and forefingers at the inside corners by the bridge of your nose. Squeeze and knead your way back and forth across your eyebrows three or four times. As they relax so do your eyes. . . . Your eyebrows will remain relaxed and will enable your eyelids to blink freely and spontaneously. . . . Feel the warmth of relaxation and circulation. . . . Finally move on to the last stage of the massage, the bony ridges around your eyes. Using your thumbs, begin at the upper indentations above the inside corners of your eyes. Do not press on your eyes themselves. Massage your way out along the bones toward the outside corners of your eyes with small, circular motions. Along the way you will encounter several more indentations. These are all acupressure points, so give them extra attention. . . . Eyes relaxing, circulation and energy flowing. . . . When you reach the outside corners of your eyes, use your index fingers to massage along the bottom bony ridge. Spend extra time on the tender spots. . . . Eyes relaxing, circulation and energy flowing. . . . When you reach the areas by your nose, reverse your direction and go back the way you came. . . . Breathe into it, and work your way back to the indentation by the bridge of your nose, changing fingers at the corners of your eyes. . . . Eyes relaxing, circulation and energy flowing. . . . Even when you are finished massaging, the relaxation, circulation, and energy will remain. . . . When you've reached that upper inside corner, keep your eyes closed while you take a moment to gently shake and relax your hands. . . . Then palm your eyes, and let them fully relax into the soothing darkness. . . . Feel the wonderful glow of relaxation and circulation throughout your back, shoulders, neck, head, face, and eyes. . . . As you relax into the darkness, the effects of your massaging sink deep into your body, mind, and visual system. . . . These positive effects are permanently a part of you now. . . . When you do open your eyes, you will find that your sight is clearer and you feel wonderfully relaxed and expansive. . . . You are seeing better and better all the time. . . . You have the power to heal your vision. . . . It's happening and you know it. . . . And it feels so very, very good. . . . In a few moments I'll count from one to five. With each number up your subconscious will more fully accept and integrate the benefits of your massage and the positive suggestions that I have made. At the same time your conscious mind will become more alert with each number up, so that by the number five you will be fully awake and alert, feeling terrific, seeing more clearly than ever before. . . . One— deepening your breathing, feeling wonderfully relaxed yet energized. Two—your energy building, your eyes, face, head, neck, shoulders, and back relaxed and comfortable. Three—halfway up. Notice how moist and relaxed your eyes feel. Four—almost all the way back. Taking deeper breaths. Feeling so good about your ever-improving vision. When you hear the next number, you'll be fully alert. Five—take in that deep breath, keep your eyes closed as you stretch and yawn. When you do open your eyes, blink softly and swing your head from side to side for a few moments. . . . Don't you feel and see wonderfully!"

o

I've had a smile on my face the whole time I've been writing this last section because I know how well everyone responds to these massages. Do your clearsighted friends a favor and share this exercise with them. All eyes, bodies, and minds benefit greatly from it. As you'll now see, it can get your whole day off to the perfect start.

During the day try to fit in at least three minisessions. During each you will be combining a brief massage with suggestions. You have a choice of just where to massage. One method is to use the back, shoulder, and neck massage for the first mini, the base of the skull and the scalp for the second, and then the forehead, jaw, and bony ridge around the eyes for the final one. This is a perfectly fine methodical approach that covers all the areas. However, I have found that many people harbor tension in certain areas more than others. They have found it beneficial to do their rapid induction and then let their awareness move around through the various possible areas that could be massaged. By doing this you can sense which area needs your attention at this point. To "sense" which spots need the massage, you simply focus your attention on them and wait patiently for an inner answer to manifest. Trust your instincts.

After you have induced your hypnosis and decided where to massage, affirm the following concepts while you massage:

o

"Relaxing, warming, letting go. . . . My eyes are relaxing right along with the muscles I am massaging. . . . Deep, soothing relaxation. . . . Circulation flowing into my eyes right along with the muscles I am massaging. . . . Everything in my visual system wonderfully relaxed. . . . The relaxation remains even when I am finished massaging. . . . Refreshed, relaxed, invigorated. . . . Circulation and energy flowing into my eyes. . . . I am ready to see clearly. . . . I know my vision is healing and improving. . . . Seeing more and more clearly every day. . . . I enjoy seeing clearly. . . ."

o

If you have time, palm for a few minutes before you count yourself up into full conscious alertness. You'll find that these brief sessions bring about an almost total recurrence of the degree of relaxation and clarity of your vision that the full session stimulated. This effect will grow as the week goes on. Your subconscious is a willing learner, and its skills improve steadily.

Later in the day your full session will be the Chinese acupressure massage. It is a powerful tonic and energizer for your entire visual system. Your eye muscles will relax as the energy is balanced and opened. When you go to sleep after this massage, your visual system will go on relaxing and balancing during the night. This is a perfect way to offset the habitual visual tension that myopes tend to display during sleep. You may also find that you enjoy adding elements of the morning massage on top of this one. If so, add them after you have finished the official session, as the suggestions are specific to the effect of acupressure.

Before you perform this massage under hypnosis, spend some time studying the illustrations on page 71 and locating the exact points on your face and around your eyes. You'll know you've found them when you experience what the Chinese call a "sour" feeling. This is a sensation that is supposed to be just short of pain, though some of the points may actually feel painful in your initial sessions. Use pressure that elicits sensation, but ease up if real pain occurs. Gentle persistence will open these energy centers, and they will gradually become more comfortable to work with.

There are four parts to this massage. The first three are single spots and the fourth is the same series of spots you rubbed along the bony ridges surrounding your eyes. You will use your thumbs to massage the first pair. They are those same indentations above the inside corners of your eyes where you began massaging the bony ridge in the previous massage. Press your thumbs into them and massage around in small, firm circular rotations.

The second spots are just in from the corners of your eyes toward the bridge of your nose. You'll use just the thumb and index finger of one hand to massage them. You may notice that this is a place you have often instinctively massaged after removing your glasses. These spots are rarely tender but feel like gristly little lumps. You will simply be rubbing in and out on these points.

The third points are sometimes the most difficult to locate, but you'll know when you've found them because they are usually the most sensitive. They are approximately one fingertip's width away from the corners of your nose. Lay your hands against your face with the top edge of your middle finger lined up with the bottom of your nose. Let your index finger lie right down next to your middle finger. Press in with it, and you should feel an indentation and the tenderness that tells you you're in the right spot. When you massage this spot, you'll want to bend your middle finger down out of the way.

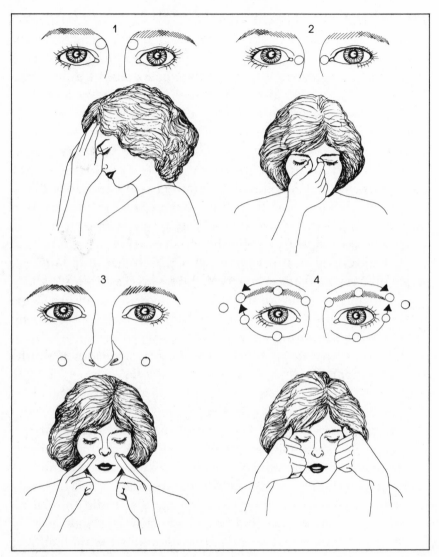

Acupressure Massage

As you can see in the illustration, the fourth part of the massage covers a number of points on those bony ridges surrounding your eyes. Rather than working each point separately, you'll be stroking across them with the knuckles of your index fingers as you bend them. Always stroke from the inside corners to the outside ones, first above your eyes and then underneath. You want to use as firm a pressure as possible without stretching the delicate skin in this area.

After your induction, this massage will take approximately sixteen minutes. You'll rub each area for about one minute while you listen to the suggestions, going over the whole procedure four times. Memorize the location and order of the points to be massaged.

After the acupressure massage there will be another brief massage that I'm sure you will also enjoy. It's amazing in that you can quite literally feel the massage in your eyes, even though you won't be touching them. In fact, you would be able to feel it even if you weren't hypnotized. You'll start by cupping your hands together, as if you were holding a baby bird in your hands. The fingertips of your right hand will rest along the edge of the thumb on your left hand, and the fingertips of your left hand will rest against the edge of the little finger of your right hand. You'll stretch your hands out flatter, palms coming close together and fingers stretching out, then round them out again, doing this over and over. And it will feel exactly as if you are actually manipulating the shape of your eyes. Eyes respond beautifully to this massage.

When you are ready, induce your hypnotic state and go on with the following:

o

"Keep your eyes closed and place your thumbs on the first points, the ones by the bridge of your nose. Begin massaging in small circular movements. Let it feel like you are breathing directly into these points as you massage them. . . . The energy within your eyes and visual system is opening and balancing. . . . As energy and circulation flow into your eyes, they relax and expand. . . . Your eyes are alive with vitality and energy. . . . Your ciliary and oblique extraocular muscles are relaxing and balancing. . . . They relax even more whenever you look into the distance. . . . They are so relaxed that your eyeballs are free to expand into a rounder shape. . . . Move on to the second points now, pressing with the thumb and index finger of one hand on the gristly spots in from the corners of your eyes. Gently massage in and out, in and out. . . . Breathe into these spots as you massage them. . . .

Energy opening, flowing, balancing. . . . Eyes relaxing and expanding. . . . Muscles relaxing and balancing. . . . Healing energy flowing into your eyes. . . . You can feel the release and the relaxation. . . . Your vision is healing and improving. . . . Move on to the third points now, pressing on the sensitive indentations along your cheekbone a finger's width from the edges of your nose. Massage in firm circular movements. . . . Healing energy is being released with each circle of your fingertips. . . . Breathe into these spots as you massage, and feel the energy flowing up into your eyes. . . . Feel it pouring into your whole visual system. . . . Circulation, energy, and relaxation opening and balancing. . . . You can feel the healing power you are releasing into your eyes. . . . Ciliary and oblique muscles relaxing, eyes expanding into a rounder shape. . . . Move on now to the last part of the massage, stroking across the bony ridges surrounding your eyes. Curl the index finger of each hand, and stroke from the inside corners out. Top, then bottom, top, then bottom. . . . As your knuckles touch each of the acupressure points, healing energy is released. Energy and circulation opening and balancing, healing your vision. . . . Muscles relaxing, eyes expanding. . . . Breathing into your eyes as you feel this massage expand them. . . . The positive effects of this released energy and relaxation remain after you are finished with the massage. . . . Releasing, relaxing, balancing, healing. . . . You are healing your vision. Your vision is improving. . . ."

At this point in the exercise, you are to go back to the beginning and repeat the massage three more times. Then go on.

"Cup your hands together now, fingertips of each hand resting against the edge of the other hand. Press down gently so that your hands flatten out more, and feel your eyes respond to this. Round your hands out again, and feel your eyes respond to this movement. Continue on this way, concentrating on the rounding movement rather than the flattening movement. Each time you round your hands, your eyes also

become rounder and shorter from front to back. Keep moving your hands and feel the massage. . . . Each time you
round your hands your eyes also become round, becoming
shorter from front to back. . . . Your eyes are changing shape,
becoming shorter from front to back. . . . Your eyes respond
beautifully, becoming rounder, and shorter from front to
back. . . . The massage feels so good. . . . Eyes massaged into
a rounder, shorter shape, and you see clearly in the distance. . . . Your eyes are relaxed, energized, and round. . . .
Your eyes coming into the shape for perfect vision in the
distance. . . . Feel them rounding. . . . Let go of the massaging action now and feel the relaxation and round shape of
your eyes. . . . Now cup your palms over your closed eyes, and
relax into the soothing darkness. . . . The energy flowing
from your palms into your eyes enhances the effects of this
massage. . . . Your ciliary and oblique muscles are wonderfully relaxed. . . . Energy flows into your eyes, and they expand into the relaxation of the muscles. . . . Your entire visual
system is soothed, relaxed, and balanced. . . . Your vision is
healing, and you see more clearly at all distances. . . . You are
ready to see clearly, and you deserve to see clearly. . . . As you
relax your eyes and visual system, they become more powerful and you see more clearly. . . . Feel the energy and the
relaxation. . . . You know your vision is improving. . . . In a
few moments I'm going to count from one to five. If you are
going to go to sleep at this time, simply let the numbers serve
as signals to deepen your relaxation, and soon you will drift
off into a deep and restful sleep, your eyes continuing to
relax and energize. If you want to come back to full conscious
alertness, the numbers will bring this awareness back while
they also reinforce your subconscious acceptance of the suggestions. . . . One—deepening your breaths, coming up relaxed and refreshed. . . . Two—feeling more awake and alert,
your eyes wonderfully relaxed and energized. . . . Three—
halfway up, noticing how moist, relaxed, and energized your
eyes feel. . . . Four—deeper breaths. Almost fully alert. Feeling confident about your ever-improving vision. When you

hear the next number bring yourself all the way back to full conscious alertness. . . . Five—all the way back. Take in a deep breath, and keep your eyes closed as you stretch and yawn. When you open them, blink softly and gently swing your head from side to side. Enjoy the relaxation and energy in your eyes and sight. . . ."

o

If you want to add massages from the morning session, now is the time to do it. By now you've experienced what an instantaneous lift to your vision massage can provide. As the week progresses you'll find that your eyes respond more and more to the massages. Many of my clients make time for massage sessions even after this stage of the program is complete. They just feel so good, and they always give that immediate lift to your visual acuity. You'll also find them useful for the alleviation of headaches and other stress reactions. Let me say it again: Massage is healing. Make it a part of your life, and give yourself this healing attention.

WEEK THREE

Dr. Bates developed the gentle exercises you'll be practicing this week. However, their effectiveness will be significantly increased by the hypnotic suggestions you will absorb while you perform them. These simple, relaxing, and yet powerful techniques are known as *long swings, sunning,* and *short swings.* They will not only increase the circulation in and relaxation of your eyes and visual system, but they will also get movement back into your vision. When tension interferes with sight, there is an actual freezing up of the visual system. The eyes are no longer able to dart about and scan over scenes for details, and their natural vibratory rhythm is shut down. These exercises will gently coax your eyes into letting go of their negative staring habits and regaining their natural movement.

The illustration on page 76 shows you how your body moves as you do the long swings. You simply stand with your feet shoulders' width apart, with the sun to your back if you are outside. Your eyes,

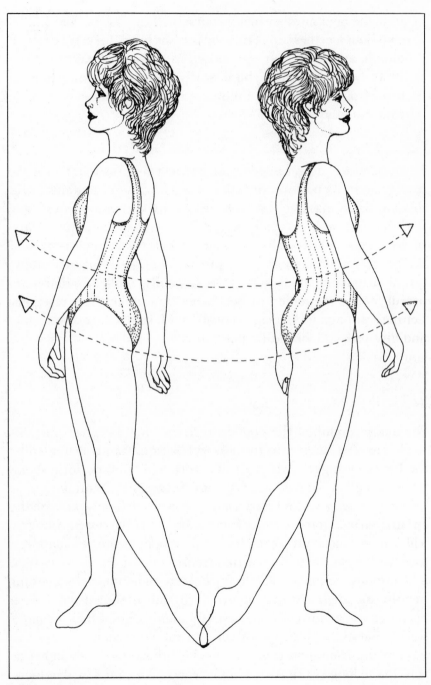

Long Swings

head, and body all move together as you swing from side to side, gently—this is not an exercise to reduce the size of your waist! Let your arms hang loosely at your sides. They will flop like limp ropes against your thighs as you swing. As you swing in one direction, let your opposite heel lift up. While swinging, remember to blink regularly, at least at the end of each swing. The ideal view to have in front of you as you swing is one where there are objects in both foreground and background. As you swing you will then experience the optical illusion of the objects at these differing distances moving in opposite directions. Swing past a window if you work indoors, as this enhances the movement. If you can arrange for soft, rhythmical music to play in the background, it will enhance the effects of these swings as well as the sunning and short swings.

Sunning is done sitting down and facing the sun or a bright light with your eyes *closed*. Be sure the angle of the light source is not so high that you have to tilt your head very far back, as this creates tension. Morning or very late afternoon sun is the best. A spotlight or floodlight is good for indoor use, but never use a heat lamp or sunlamp. You'll simply be swinging your head across the sun or light in a variety of directions, up and down, back and forth, diagonally, and in circles. The sun will soothe and warm your eye and neck muscles and help them relax more into the swinging movement. You won't be spending more than a few minutes in the direct sunlight, but use a sunscreen if you are worried about the effects of ultraviolet light. Sunlight is not only relaxing but it emits healthy waves of light that benefit us emotionally and physically. If you use a light instead of the sun, activate your powers of imagination and let it seem like actual sunlight. Keep the word "sun" in your suggestion even if you use a light. The idea of the healing power of the sun will enhance the effectiveness of the artificial light.

The short swings involve some of the same moves as the sunning exercise but are performed facing away from the sun or light. With them you will be visualizing movement across imagined black lines. The movement will loosen your eyes and the visualization will improve this skill necessary for clear vision. Each phase will take about five minutes, plus the induction beforehand and palming time afterward. Induce your hypnosis and then follow these instructions:

o

"Palm your eyes, and feel them relax into the darkness. This deep relaxation readies them for the long swings, sunning, and short swings you are about to perform. These exercises will have a profound loosening and balancing effect on your eyes and visual system. Your eyes will not only relax and balance, but they will also regain their natural vibratory rhythm. During the exercises you will remain in a pleasant, deep state of hypnosis, yet your mind and body will respond accurately and alertly to all the positive suggestions made. Your balance will be steady when you stand up and do the long swings. Your eyes will remain relaxed and will respond effortlessly and naturally to all the suggestions made. . . . Let your breath seem to flow directly into your eyes, and feel them let go with each exhalation. . . . Relax your hands down from your eyes now. Let your eyes remain closed as you begin to swing or roll your head gently from side to side. . . . Now open your eyes and blink softly as you continue swinging your head for a few more moments. . . . Stand up now and position yourself with your feet shoulders' width apart, facing away from the sun and looking out at the view around you. Begin swinging lazily from side to side, arms hanging loosely at your sides. As you swing in each direction, let the opposite heel lift off the ground. Blink your eyes softly, at least at the end of each swing, and let your eyes, head, and body all move together. Allow your eyes to slide over the view as you swing past it. . . . Let everything slide by as you swing past. . . . Relaxed, easy breaths as you swing. . . . If there is a foreground as well as a background in the view you are sliding, be aware that the background moves with you and the foreground objects seem to be sliding by in the opposite direction. If there is only a background in the distance, notice that it moves in the opposite direction of your swing. . . . Let the world slide by. . . . With each swing your eyes relax more. . . . Ciliary and oblique muscles letting go, eyes expanding. . . . Seeing clearer and clearer as you swing, blink, and breathe. . . . The swinging motion has a massaging effect on your eyes. . . . Natural, effortless movement returning to your eyes and visual system. . . . Natural movement and vibration returning to your eyes. . . . Take a moment to feel this movement and vibration as you swing. Close one eye and very gently touch your eyelid with one finger. You can feel the eye vibrating and moving. . . . Take your finger away, open the eye again, and keep on swinging. . . . Energy and movement are natural to your vision now. . . . Breathe, blink, swing, and let the world slide by. . . . Your eyes relaxing and your vision clearing with each and every swing. . . . A pleasant letting go and sense of freedom spreading throughout your eyes, visual system, face, neck, and shoulders as you swing. . . . It feels good to let the world swing by. . . . Details flash in clearly as you slide by them. . . . Eyes relaxing, aligning, balancing. . . . The side-to-side motion massages your eye muscles. As they relax, your eyes expand and become rounder and you see more clearly in the distance. . . . Easy, effortless swings. Let the world slide by as your vision relaxes. . . . Clear details jump out at you as you slide over them. . . . Movement and vibration are again a part of your visual skills. . . . Muscles relaxed, eyes rounder, you see more clearly in the distance. . . . Let the swinging motion gradually subside now. . . . Blink softly and look around you, feeling the life and relaxation in your vision, seeing more clearly than before. . . . Sit down now, facing the sun or a bright light with your eyes *closed*. . . . Relax into the soothing warmth penetrating through your closed lids and into your eyes. . . . In a moment I'll count down from three to one. With each number down feel yourself sinking down into deeper and deeper relaxation. Three—letting go, sinking down. Two—deeper down, more relaxed. One—way down, completely relaxed. . . . With your eyes still closed and your face to the sun, now feel its warmth relaxing your eyes even more. Relax into the soothing warmth of the sun. You are absorbing the healing warmth and energy of the sun. . . . Feel that you are breathing this healing energy into your eyes and visual system. . . . Warming, relaxing, energizing, healing. . . . Now begin gently swinging your head from left to right, back and forth across the sun. . . . Notice that as you swing in one direction the sun seems to move in the opposite direction. . . . Breathe as you swing. . . . Enjoy the apparent opposite movement of the sun. . . . With every easy swing your eyes, face, neck, and shoulders relax more and more. . . . Your eyes seem to float along with the swinging motion, feeling loose and massaged. . . . Ciliary and oblique muscles letting go, eyes becoming expanded and rounder. . . . It feels good to relax into the sun's warmth as you swing across it. . . . Vibration and movement restored to your eyes. . . . Your vision is improving, you feel it and you know it. . . . Change the direction of your swing now to an up-and-down movement over the sun. . . . Neck muscles relaxing as you move your head gently up and down. The sun appearing to move in the opposite direction of your swing. It moves up when you bend your head down. It moves down when you lift your head up. . . . Breathe as you swing. . . . Ciliary and oblique muscles relaxing, eyes expanding and rounding. . . . Energy and movement returning to your vision. . . . Eye muscles relaxing, aligning, balancing. . . . The movement and the sun's warmth and energy healing your vision. . . . Relaxing and loosening with each up-and-down swing. . . . It feels so good as your shoulders, neck, face, and eyes relax into this movement and the warmth of the sun. . . . The sun appears to move in the opposite direction of your swings. . . . The optic center of your brain at the base of your skull is being massaged and energized by the up-and-down swinging motion of your head. . . . You are ready to see clearly, you can feel the changes taking place. . . . Change the direction of your swing now to a diagonal movement, kitty-corner up to the left and down to the right. The sun moves in the opposite direction of your swing. Your neck muscles relax more and more. . . . Eye muscles relaxing, balancing, aligning. . . . Eyes expanding to a rounder shape. . . . Up to the left, down to the right, relaxing into the soothing warmth of the sun. . . . Neck, shoulders, optic center, and eyes loosening and relaxing. . . . With every swing of your head your vision is healing. . . . Breathe as you swing. . . . Looser and looser. . . . Energy and circulation flowing into your eyes and visual system. . . . Change the direction of your swing to the other diagonal now, up to the right and down to the left. . . . Breathing and swinging. . . . Muscles relaxing. . . . Eye muscles loosening, balancing, aligning. . . . Feel the gently penetrating warmth and healing energy of the sun as you swing by it. The sun appears to move in the opposite direction of your swing. . . . As your ciliary and oblique muscles relax, your eyes expand and round. . . . Shoulder and neck muscles softening, optic center massaged by the movement of your head. . . . Energy and vibration returning to your eyes. . . . Your vision is improving, and you know it. . . . Let the diagonal movement subside and begin making circles around the sun in a clockwise direction. Nice, easy looping circles. . . . Smoothly around and around. . . . Neck and shoulders relaxing, optic center being massaged. . . . Eye muscles relaxing, balancing, aligning. . . . Breathe as you circle around the sun. . . . Soak in the soothing warmth and energy of the sun as you circle around it. . . . Circulation opening and flowing freely. . . . Looser and looser. . . . Face and eye muscles wonderfully relaxed. . . . Reverse the direction of your circles now and go around the sun counterclockwise. . . . Breathing easily, moving freely. . . . Neck and shoulders relaxing while your optic center is massaged. . . . Eye muscles relaxing, balancing, aligning. . . . The sun's healing warmth and energy flowing into you. Breathe it in. Feel it relaxing and healing your vision. . . . Easy looping circles. . . . So wonderfully relaxed. . . . Everything relaxed, balanced, and aligned. . . . Your vision is improving and you know it. . . . Now let the motion gradually stop. Feel how your neck and head float in comfort above your shoulders. Feel the relaxation in your neck and eyes. . . . Cover your closed eyes with your palms for a few moments. Feel how they now relax into the soothing darkness. . . . This brief rest in the darkness allows your eyes and visual system to fully absorb and integrate the affects of the sunning swings. . . . Feel your eyes relaxing more deeply with each of your easy breaths out. . . . As much as they are relaxed already, they will now let go even more with each number that I count down from three to one. Three—a deep letting go. Two—feel that pleasant sinking sensation. One—completely relaxed. . . . Natural relaxation, energy, and vibration are restored to your eyes and visual system. All the interconnected muscles from your shoulders, neck, and face to your eyes are relaxed, balanced, and aligned. They work in harmony with each other to allow you clear vision at all distances. . . . In a few moments you will begin moving these muscles into even deeper relaxation at the same time that you develop your power of visualization that will further improve your vision. . . . Facing *away* from the sun, keep your eyes *closed* and relax your hands down. . . . Imagine that there is a shiny, white three-by-five card suspended about five feet away directly in front of you. To this image add a dark, glossy black line drawn vertically down the middle of the card. Be aware of the contrast between the white and the black. Now add two black dots into the image, each in the center of one half of the card, the black line in between them. In reality move your head and eyes so that they are pointed directly at the imaginary black dot on the right side of the line. Now move your head and eyes to the left as you imagine looking at that black dot. Swing back and forth from dot to dot, across the black line. As you imagine swinging past the line, it will appear to move in the opposite direction. Breathe and swing from dot to dot, remaining aware of the opposite movement of the line. . . . You can easily imagine the sharp contrast between the black and the white. . . . With each easy, short swing of your head, your eyes relax more and more. . . . Your eyes feel like they are floating, feel like they are being massaged. . . . The apparent movement of the black line in the opposite direction of your swing dramatically increases the energy and vibration within your eyes. . . . Shoulders, neck, head, and eyes relaxed. . . . Eyes becoming rounder. . . . You can clearly visualize the white card, black line, black dots, and the movement of the line as you swing your head from dot to dot. . . . Let go now of the swinging and the image. Feel the energy and relaxation in your eyes. . . . Now imagine another white card in the same place in space. Give it a shiny black horizontal line across the center from left to right. Above and below the line, in the center of each half, add a black dot. Begin swinging your head up and down now, from dot to dot, aware that the line moves in the opposite direction of your swing. . . . The card is very white, the dots and line are very black. . . . You can easily, clearly visualize this image. . . . Eyes relaxing and energizing as you swing from dot to dot. . . . You can feel the relaxation and the energy. . . . Aligning, balancing, relaxing, energizing. . . . Your sight is improving. You know it and it feels good. . . . Shoulders, neck, and optic center massaged as you swing from dot to dot. . . . Eyes wonderfully loose, relaxed, and expanded. . . . Let go of the movement and the visualization now. Change your position if you wish, and palm your eyes. . . . Feel them relax into the darkness. . . . Breathe into them, and feel them let go more with each breath out. . . . Wonderfully, deeply relaxed. . . . The swings and visualizations have relaxed, balanced, and energized your eyes and your vision has improved. . . . Your eyes are relaxed and rounder and have learned new, positive habits of vision. . . . Your eyes vibrate with natural rhythm and scan scenes rapidly for detail. . . . You blink often, spontaneously, and effortlessly. You are ready for clear vision, and your eyes and visual system cooperate. You see more clearly all the time. . . . Your vision is improving. You know it, you feel it, and it feels good. . . . In a few moments I'm going to count from one to five. At the subconscious level each number up will reinforce all the positive changes you've achieved within your eyes and visual system. At the conscious level the numbers will serve as reminders that it's time now to return to full alertness. . . . One—deepening your breathing. Confident of your ever-improving vision. . . . Two—come up. Feeling the vibration and relaxation in your eyes. . . . Three—halfway up. Your eyes feel so moist and relaxed. . . . Four—deeper breathing.

Feeling wonderfully refreshed in every way, especially in your vision. When you hear the last number bring yourself all the way up. Five—a deep breath in, keep your eyes closed as you stretch and yawn. Fully alert. When you open your eyes, swing your head from side to side and blink softly. . . . Enjoy your new visual skills and the deeper relaxation of your eyes."

o

Just like the massages, these exercises will increase in effectiveness during the week. Not only will your vision be more clear but you'll also experience a new vitality in your eyes. The release of that vibratory rhythm will give you a sense of freedom and expansion both emotionally and visually.

During your minisessions you will not be doing any actual swinging or sunning. The suggestions will reinforce what happens during the full sessions as well as deeper acceptance of all the changes you have been bringing about within your vision.

After inducing your hypnosis, confirm the following ideas to yourself, palming as you do so:

o

"My eyes are wonderfully relaxed and energized. . . . Every time I swing, sun, and visualize my vision improves. . . . My eyes are lively and scan scenes for details. . . . My ciliary and oblique muscles are relaxed. . . . My eyes relax and become even rounder whenever I look into the distance. . . . My shoulders, neck, head, and facial muscles remain relaxed. . . . Everything in my visual system cooperates so that I see more clearly. . . . I am ready for clear vision. . . . I deserve clear vision. . . . My sight is improving all the time. . . . It all feels so very good. . . ."

o

Count yourself up while reaffirming your relaxed, clear vision and your mental alertness.

By this time, if not before, you will most likely be experiencing occasional moments that we call "clear flashes." These are precisely what they sound like, moments when everything is suddenly crystal clear. They won't last too long initially, but they will last longer and become more frequent as your work continues. Clarity is something new to your visual system, so it pops back into the old, familiar habits. Gradually it will get used to the new habits and the changes will become permanent. In the meantime, simply appreciate these demonstrations of your real visual ability. On the other hand, some people progress gradually without ever experiencing clear flashes. We're all different; your system is finding its own individual way of changing.

WEEK FOUR

This week concentrates on developing your visualization powers. Dr. Bates discovered that when people could learn to visualize well, they then saw clearly. It's no coincidence that most myopes have trouble visualizing. However, once this limitation is overcome, visual progress is rapid. The brief imaging experiences you have had so far in the program have primed your visual system to expand now into greater expertise at visualizing. Just like an athlete increases his or her athletic skill by repeatedly imagining performing flawlessly, so you will improve your outer vision by developing it at the inner level.

One of your full sessions will involve visualizing real scenes, while the other is more symbolic and geared toward the physical healing of your eyes. The "real" scenes are set in nature and are emotionally as well as visually refreshing. I have laid out the scripts so that you begin your day with this inspiring experience. However, some of my clients with stress-producing jobs have found that they prefer this visual vacation as a way to unwind from their day. If this is the case for you, feel free to reverse the order of the sessions.

If your initial attempts at visualizing aren't as successful as you'd like, just remember that visualizing is another learned skill that takes time to perfect. You may also simply be getting in your own way by expecting too much. A movie screen is not going to leap up under your eyelids and produce vivid images. Visualizing is a little like sleep; you can't achieve it by trying to force it to come. Just relax and think about the scenes you'll hear being described. It's like reading a book. Once you become immersed in the story, images of it start coming to you. Then, after you are able to practice seeing clearly mentally, you will be able to transfer this skill into actual seeing.

For your first daily session, hypnotize yourself, palm your eyes, and then immerse yourself in the following fantasy:

○

"Your eyes are wonderfully, deeply relaxed. They and your entire visual system will respond to the following images as if they were real. Seeing this clearly with your mind's eye will enable your physical eyes to function with the same skilled clarity. . . . Think what it would be like to wake up in the morning on the deck of your own private yacht or ship. Your eyes are not yet open, but you can feel the gentle rolling of the boat on the water. You can smell the salt spray in the air. You can feel the gently penetrating rays of the morning sun on your body. You feel wonderful, glad to be alive, and filled with well-being. . . . Imagine opening your eyes and looking up at the clear blue sky above you. One fleecy white cloud is drifting by. A seagull flies overhead, and you can hear its cry as you observe its white feathers and orange beak. It's free and beautiful as it floats through the air. You feel that same freedom within yourself. . . . Now it's time to get up, feeling refreshed, and look around you. What kind of a ship are you on? Is it a motor yacht or a sailing ship? It's your boat, you can imagine it any way you want to. Observe all the details. . . . Now look beyond your ship. You are floating on clear aquamarine water just off the coast of a lush tropical island. The water is so clear you can see a dolphin in its depths. The dolphin shoots to the surface, breaks out of the water, and grins at you in welcome. You feel welcome, and you enjoy watching her as she plays in the water. . . . Looking toward shore, you watch the waves crest and break and their white foam flow onto the beach. The sand on the beach is pristine white, sparkling in the morning sun. Beyond the beach is a magnificent, green tropical jungle, the foliage rich and lush. You see palm trees with coconuts hanging from them and vines and bushes with brightly colored flowers. Perched high atop one palm tree is a parrot with brilliant blue and yellow feathers. As you view this scene, your eyes are relaxed and your vision is clear. . . . You feel wonderfully relaxed and at peace with yourself and the world. . . . The dolphin still swims nearby and seems to be beckoning you to join her. Why not? The water is warm, clear, and inviting. So you dive in, relishing the feel of the water against your skin. Its saltiness tastes good. The dolphin comes to greet you, and you stroke her cool, slippery skin. Again you feel welcome. Together you and the dolphin dive deep beneath the water where you swim among beds of coral of pink, white, and lavender. Brightly colored tropical fish come to greet you, not in the least bit afraid. One of them nibbles your fingers in a gentle hello. Swim and play here beneath the ocean's surface. . . . Finally you decide to swim to shore. The fish and the dolphin accompany you as you swim with strong but effortless strokes. Soon you can stand on the ocean floor, and you say good-bye to the dolphin and the fish before walking in toward shore. . . . The air is warmer now, and you can feel the sun drying you as you begin to emerge from the water. The wet sand has felt good under your feet, but it is pleasant to feel the warmth of the dry sand as you reach the beach. . . . Let your gaze follow the shoreline into the distance. Your eyes relax as you look into the distance. You clearly see a small flock of water birds dipping their beaks into the wet sand as the waves go out. . . . Looking at the jungle, you see an inviting opening leading into the foliage. Next to the opening is a large rock. On it are clothes. They are for you to wear. As you walk to the rock, still feeling the warm sand beneath your feet, you see the color and style of the clothing. Like the ship, they are your own and you can let them be any way you like. When you reach them, examine them more thoroughly and feel their texture. Go through the process of dressing, enjoying the feeling of the cloth against your skin. . . . Once dressed, it's time to move on to another beautiful place. The path through the tropical rain forest is friendly and inviting. As you walk along it, you enjoy the gorgeous tropical foliage. The sun filters through the leaves, lighting your way. There is soft moss beneath your feet. Here and there you see orchids and other flowers among the leaves. You stop to smell one and relish its sweet scent. . . . You feel carefree and confident as you walk on, enjoying the sights around you. Then you see bright light at the end of the jungle trail. When you reach the opening, you realize you have come to another climatic zone. You have come to the edge of a mountain meadow on a warm spring day. The air smells of pine needles. The meadow is ringed with pine trees, and you can see the pinecones clearly. In the distance is a snowcapped mountain peak, towering majestically as it reaches into the brilliant blue sky above. Above the mountaintop floats one puffy white cloud. A bald eagle soars by near the cloud, and you can see its white head in contrast to its brown body glistening almost gold in the sunlight. . . . As you look back down at the meadow, you can smell the sweetness of the lush grass. The grass is dotted with wildflowers of red, pink, yellow, and blue. . . . At the opposite edge of the meadow you see two deer, a doe and her spotted fawn. They regard you peacefully with their warm, brown eyes, seeming to welcome you to their meadow. A brown rabbit hops out of the bushes near the deer and nibbles at the grass. You can see his whiskers and his twitching nose as he sits up and smells the air, still chewing on a blade of grass. Then with an exuberant kick of his hind legs, he bounds back into the underbrush. You look to a tree near the grazing deer and see a gray squirrel placing a nut into a hole in the bark. His fluffy tail twitches in excitement. Looking back down at the meadow's edge, you see a mother skunk appear, followed by three babies in single file. They pass by the deer and back into the forest. . . . You feel very much at home here in this beautiful place. Perhaps you'd like to walk out into the meadow and explore it more closely. Perhaps you'd like to run free like the animals. Smell the flowers, roll in the grass, do whatever you'd like. Just be aware of how wonderful it is to be alive and to see so clearly. . . . In addition to feeling yourself in this scene, you can see yourself in it, as if from a distance. You look radiantly healthy, carefree, and relaxed. You know you see clearly. . . . Let the images fade now and just relax into the darkness once again. . . . Recognize how wonderfully relaxed and energized you feel, physically, emotionally, and visually. These feelings will remain with you. Well-being and clear vision are within you and will continue as a simple matter of course. . . . In a few moments I will count from one to five. With each number up your visual system will even more fully integrate its skill at seeing clearly. At the same time the numbers will signal your conscious mind that it's time to return to full alertness. . . . One—coming up, feeling terrific, knowing you see clearly. Two—breaths continuing to deepen, your visual system understanding how to function clearly. Three—halfway up. Notice how refreshed and moist your eyes feel. Four—almost all the way back. So confident in your improving vision. Come all the way back up when you hear the next number. Five—a deep breath and a stretch, keeping your eyes closed for a few more moments. Completely alert. When you open your eyes, roll your head from side to side and blink softly. Enjoy the clarity of your vision."

o

As you progress through the week with this visualization, you may find yourself spontaneously adding images to those presented. That's fine. Embellish the format any way you wish. Conversely, if there are images that you do not find pleasing, go ahead and change them to something you like. Chances are you've never had a bad experience with a deer, but some people do have unpleasant associations with the ocean and the beach. If this is the case with you, make up another scene as a substitute. Just be sure to give yourself lots of details, from colors to textures to smells. All of our senses work together, so your vision receives stimulation even when you are imagining something entirely different.

Your minisessions this week will not involve actual visualizations, but they will reinforce your ability to visualize as well as other important concepts you have already learned.

For the minis, use your rapid induction, palm your eyes, and repeat the following ideas over and over to yourself:

o

"My eyes are wonderfully, deeply relaxed. . . . My sight is improving. . . . I visualize effortlessly and clearly. . . . Whenever I visualize my eyes and visual system function as if I were seeing in reality. My ciliary and extraocular oblique muscles relax when I look into the distance, and I see clearly. . . . I am ready to see clearly. I deserve to see clearly. . . . The optic center of my brain directs my eyes to see clearly, and it interprets images it receives as clear. . . . I visualize clearly and I see clearly. . . . I am confident that my vision is improving, and it feels good."

o

Although, as I've mentioned, you may choose to reverse the order of the long sessions this week, I have placed the following one last for good reason. It will focus on physiological changes in your eyes and improved functioning of your whole visual system. Doing this just before you go to sleep allows your subconscious to go right on effecting the changes you have been focusing upon. With this in mind, I have again included the option of drifting off to sleep when the session is done. But, of course, change this direction if it doesn't apply to your situation. If you do choose to go to sleep after the healing visualization session, you might want to look into a technique known as lucid dreaming. There is an excellent book of the same name (*Lucid Dreaming* by Stephen LaBerge [Los Angeles: J. P. Tarcher, 1985]). One of my clients applied lucid dreaming to this session, and after a week of dreaming about the changes occurring she showed a remarkable improvement.

Once again, induce your hypnotic state, palm your eyes, and let the following suggestions soak in:

o

"Let your eyes melt into relaxation behind your palms. . . .
Breathe into your eyes. Feel them expand with each breath in
and relax with each breath out. . . . They relax more with
each easy breath out. . . . As your ciliary and oblique muscles
relax, your eyes have room to expand into a rounder shape.
Shorter and rounder from front to back than before. . . . Feel
how much more relaxed your eyes are already. . . . Now create
a visual image of your eyes. See your lenses and the ciliary
muscles attached to them. See those oblique extraocular
muscles around your eyes. Let yourself see and feel some
tightness in these muscles. See and feel the constriction in
your lenses and eyeballs caused by these tight muscles. . . .
Now imagine a pair of hands coming into this picture. These
are healing hands that will massage your muscles into complete relaxation. See them first kneading and massaging your
oblique muscles. As you see the muscles respond to this healing touch and relax, feel the relaxation as well. . . . It feels so
good to have those muscles massaged. You can feel relaxation, circulation, and energy flowing into them. . . . Deep,
healing massage. . . . The muscles letting go and relaxing. . . . Letting go and relaxing. . . . Softening under the
healing touch. . . . Softening under the healing touch. . . .
So deeply, wonderfully relaxed. . . . Relaxed yet vibrantly
alive. . . . See those hands, feel that massage. . . . Be aware
that as these oblique muscles are softening and letting go,
your eyeballs have room to expand into a rounder shape.
Rounder, and shorter from front to back. . . . They feel alive
and free . . . free to round out . . . free to see clearly. . . . Now
let the healing hands move on to your ciliary muscles.
Smaller, thinner, but just as tight as your obliques were before
the massage. They are holding your lenses in a tight, concave
shape. . . . But they immediately begin to relax as the hands
massage them. . . . Responding beautifully, stretching and
relaxing. . . . Becoming softer and softer. . . . As they soften

and stretch out, your lenses are able to relax into a more convex shape, round like your eyes. . . . See and feel it happening. . . . It feels so good. . . . Relaxation and circulation flowing into your ciliary muscles and your lenses. . . . The tight, concave lenses created additional pressure within your eyes that helped keep them too elongated. Now that pressure is released, and your eyes are even more free to come into a nice round shape. . . . Your eyes are shorter than before from front to back, the perfect shape for clear vision at all distances. . . . Ciliary muscles relaxed, lenses resting in a convex shape. . . . Let the image fade away, and enjoy the feelings of health and relaxation in your eyes, lenses, ciliary and oblique muscles. . . . Go back to feeling your breath flow into your eyes. . . . Now add the image of color to this feeling. Your breath is energy. See that energy as a golden light, pouring into your eyes. . . . This energy expands and further relaxes your eyes. . . . They are relaxed but alive with golden glowing energy. . . . This energy also stimulates the rods and cones of your retinas. . . . Because of this energization, your rods and cones are more capable than ever before of recording clear images. . . . Feel the golden light penetrating and stimulating your retinas. . . . Now let the golden energy flow out through your optic nerves and into the optic center of your brain. . . . This control tower of your vision is energized and its powers increased. . . . Because of this healing energization, the optic center of your brain is able to send out better instructions to your eyes for clear vision, and it is more skilled at interpreting images clearly. . . . See your whole visual system glowing with golden light, the muscles, the lenses, the eyeballs, the retinas, the optic nerves, the optic center of your brain. . . . Glowing golden with healing energy. . . . You can feel the energy vibrating everywhere in your visual system. . . . It feels so good to release this healing power. . . . Everything in your visual system is able to function better than ever before. . . . Let the image fade now, but continue to feel its healing effects. . . . Relaxed, energized, healed. . . . This whole process will continue within your visual system. . . . In a few moments I'll begin counting from one to five. If you would like to go to sleep now, simply let the numbers and suggestions serve as signals to relax you into a deep and restful sleep. Otherwise, let them bring your conscious mind back to full alertness while your subconscious even more fully accepts the healing you have accomplished. . . . One—deepening your breathing. Coming up relaxed and refreshed. . . . Two—more alert with each breath in. Eyes feeling so relaxed and healed. . . . Three—halfway up. Feel the energy and moisture in your eyes. . . . Four—deeper breaths, almost all the way back. So completely confident that the power of your mind is healing your vision. Come all the way back when you hear the next number. . . . Five—a deep breath, a stretch and a yawn, leave your eyes closed as you take down your hands. When you do open them, roll or swing your head gently from side to side and blink your eyes softly. Accept your own healing power."

o

The healing power of imagery is profound. During this week I'm sure you will be more and more pleased with your increasing powers of visualization and the results they bring. Like so many other elements of the HypnoVision program, this is another that you can add to your daily life well after the time you spend working on your vision. Anything you can visualize yourself doing well is something you can bring into reality.

WEEK FIVE

Now you're ready to put all this groundwork to use in some directed seeing. You've been building visual skills; now you will expand on those you have and put them to work. In the past, people working on their vision constantly had to remember consciously to use proper habits of vision. You won't have to worry about that because the instructions for correctly using your eyes will be imbedded at the subconscious level. After this week you will automatically use your eyes in the most efficient and effective manner.

It was Dr. Bates who first realized that there were positive and negative habits of vision. Eyes that see clearly scan over scenes for bits of detail, move freely and spontaneously, blink with gentle regularity, and are aided in their efforts by unconstricted breathing. When there is stress in the visual system, everything freezes up. The eyes lose not only their natural vibration but also the scanning movement that accompanies this vibration. Tightness in the eyelids cuts off the natural blinking response, and the resulting dryness in the corneas further inhibits clear sight. Constricted breathing cuts off circulation to the eyes and maintains the cycle of tension.

When I first began using hypnosis in vision work, I thought that the exercises for relearning proper habits of vision could be bypassed by direct suggestions about picking up details, blinking, and breathing, such as the ones you've already been using. This worked for some people, but the effect was generally not what I had hoped for. However, training the eyes to work properly while under hypnosis did the trick. When you actually practice, these skills are rapidly incorporated into and remembered by the subconscious. By the end of this week you'll be using your eyes as you were meant to.

I have referred to the scanning movement of the eyes, but a more basic skill precedes it in visual training. We call it *edging*. Bates discovered that the eyes best recovered their natural movement when the eyes and the head moved together as a unit and when objects viewed were first outlined by the eyes before moving into the finer details. You'll find it easy to keep your head moving with your eyes if you think of your nose as the leader. Let your nose do the outlining edging of objects and your eyes will follow along in an easy, relaxed manner.

Myopes are notoriously unobservant, even with their glasses on. By practicing memorizing the scenes around you, you will also be teaching your eyes to become alert gatherers of visual information. In the last week your visualization powers increased, and this week they will expand further by learning *really* to take in the details around you. This will have a strong positive impact on your visual acuity.

As in the first week, you will repeat the same full session twice a day. During it you will be observing your immediate surroundings.

Your own living room will probably be fine, but if your decorations and furniture are on the sparse side it would be good to add to them. This is a great time for vases with flowers, new pictures, new knickknacks. You want to have plenty of things to look at. When clients come to my home for their sessions, they do this exercise out in my yard, which boasts lots of colorful plants and a magnificent view of the surrounding countryside. They all learn this landscape by heart while their visual system learns how to function in all situations.

So make your surroundings as interesting as possible, induce your hypnosis, and then follow the directions in this script:

o

"Palm your eyes and feel them relax into the soothing darkness. . . . Your entire visual system is wonderfully relaxed. Your oblique and ciliary muscles, your retinas, the optic center of your brain, your eyelids, your face, head, neck, and shoulders—all completely relaxed. . . . Your eyes are balanced, aligned, and supported by all your extraocular muscles. . . . Your eyes are relaxed yet energized. Breathe into your eyes and feel them pulsate with vitality and energy. . . . You are ready to see clearly. . . . All the work you have already done with your eyes has readied them to learn quickly and fully the proper habits of vision. . . . When it is time to use your eyes during this session, they will remain relaxed and energized. When you look into the distance, your ciliary and oblique muscles will relax even more. As you take in the view around you, you will first edge the outlines of the largest objects as if you were drawing around them with your nose. Your eyes, head, and neck will move as a coordinated unit. You will then scan all over the objects, still following your nose, and pick up even more details. As you observe what is around you, you will breathe evenly and blink frequently. Everything in your visual system will work together as a coordinated team to bring you clear vision. . . . You are interested in everything around you, and you enjoy picking out visual details. . . . Relax your palms down from your eyes.

Keep your eyes closed for a few moments as they adjust to the
light coming in through your closed lids. You are ready to see
clearly. . . . Remaining in your relaxed hypnotic state of
mind, open your eyes, blink softly, and swing your head
gently from side to side. . . . Sit with a relaxed but straight
spine, your neck and head lifted above your shoulders, your
chin pulled a little in as opposed to your jaw jutting out. As
you look around you, let your nose be the leader. Breathe
evenly and blink softly as you take in the scene around
you. . . . Be aware of the largest shapes within your view. If
you are inside, the walls are the largest shapes. Point your
nose at a spot on the outer edge of the largest object you can
see. Edge around it as if there were a long, telescoping pencil
attached to the end of your nose. Outline it several times in
one direction and then go back around it in the opposite
direction. . . . Breathing and blinking as you edge. As you
move, blink, and breathe, the details become more clear. . . .
You are aware of and interested in the colors and shapes that
you see. . . . Take your time, edge leisurely. . . . After you have
thoroughly edged this object, begin scanning it for details.
Follow your nose and swing your head as you scan. Breathe
and blink. Whenever your scanning brings you to a new
detail, edge it. Notice shapes, colors, and even textures. . . .
As you edge and scan, your visual system understands that
its job is to pick up and record these details. . . . Working
from the largest to the smallest, systematically edge and scan
everything in your view. . . . Breathing and blinking and following your nose. Nice easy movements. . . . Movement is a
natural and effortless part of your visual skills. . . . You are
interested in picking out all the details in this scene. . . . You
enjoy noticing details. . . . Your sight is relaxed yet active and
energetic. . . . Breathing, blinking, scanning, and edging. . . .
Your sight is becoming clearer and clearer as you scan and
edge your way through the scene around you. . . . Always
edge around objects and details in both directions. . . . Movement is natural to your vision and brings you clear vision. . . .
Your eyes are carried along by the movement of your head.

The movement has a massaging effect on your eyes. They continue to relax. Your ciliary and oblique muscles relax as you look into the distance. . . . You are aware of colors as well as details, and the colors seem very vivid. . . . Breathing, blinking, scanning, and edging. . . . Your neck relaxes as you scan and edge for details. . . . Now begin swinging your head from left to right, back and forth over the view in front of you. Keep the movement going and simply be aware of the color red. As you swing your head, anything that is red will seem to jump out at you as you swing by it. . . . Your eyes and your brain are working together so that you are very aware of the color red whenever you swing by it. . . . Now be aware of the color blue. All the blue objects in your view will seem to jump out as you swing by them. Breathing and blinking as you swing from side to side. . . . Blue stands out among all the colors you swing by. . . . Now be aware of the color yellow as you swing. . . . All the yellows pop out as you swing your head and eyes gently from side to side. . . . Breathing and blinking. . . . Breathing and blinking are a natural part of your visual system. . . . Movement is a natural part of your visual system. . . . Now be aware of the color green as you swing. . . . The greens stand out vividly as you swing by them. . . . Your eyes continuing to loosen as you swing. . . . Ciliary and oblique muscles relax as you swing. . . . Be aware of green as you swing. . . . Your sight is observant and spontaneous. . . . Now edge and scan your way around your view again. You may notice that you see even more details than before. . . . Feel the freedom and movement in your sight. . . . Edge windows, doors, plants, whatever is in your scene. . . . Breathing and blinking. . . . Interested in all the details. . . . Eyes moist and relaxed. . . . Now close your eyes. Remember what you have been looking at. Remember the largest objects and work your way down to the smallest. Where are they in relationship to other objects? Remember the colors, the shapes, the textures. . . . See the whole scene clearly in your mind's eye. . . . Your power of visualization is strong and you clearly remember what you have seen. . . . Now open your eyes again, blinking softly. Any details and objects that you forgot about will jump out at you. Edge them, add them to your visual inventory. . . . Breathing, blinking, moving. . . . Close your eyes again, and once more remember what you have seen. . . . You have a good visual memory, and it aids in the clarity of your vision. . . . You remember colors and shapes and details. . . . You see and visualize clearly. . . . As you visualize what you have seen, you can feel your eyes moving over the scene as they remember it. . . . Open your eyes once more and look around you, breathing, blinking, and observing any other details that you might have missed. . . . Every time you do this exercise, your entire visual system more fully incorporates movement, breathing, blinking, and the ability to pick up details. Seeing more clearly all the time. . . . Close your eyes now and palm them. . . . Feel your eyes let go into the soothing darkness. . . . Your eyes and visual system have learned to see with clear, relaxed spontaneity. Movement of your eyes and head is natural and effortless. You breathe and blink as you see. . . . It is natural and effortless for you to keep your eyes moving. . . . You scan and edge scenes for detail. . . . Your ciliary and oblique muscles relax as you look into the distance. . . . You are interested in observing details. . . . Your eyes and visual system are alive with relaxation and energy. . . . You feel good about the positive changes in your vision. . . . You are seeing more clearly all the time. . . . You deserve clear vision and you are ready for it. . . . The visual center of your brain understands how to direct your eyes to see clearly. . . . The visual center of your brain clearly interprets the images sent to it. . . . Your vision is improving and you know it. . . . It feels so good to see more clearly. . . . In a few moments I'm going to begin counting from one to five. At the subconscious level each of these numbers will allow your visual system to integrate even more fully everything it has learned. At the conscious level these numbers will serve as reminders to come back to full waking alertness. One—coming up, breaths deepening. Feeling rested and refreshed. Two—so very confident of your ever-improving vision.

Three—halfway up, your eyes feeling moist and refreshed. Four—almost all the way back. Your eyes and brain now able to function in perfect coordination. Come all the way back when you hear the next number. Five—a deep breath and a stretch as you remove your hands from your closed eyes. Alert, confident, and refreshed. When you open your eyes, blink softly and swing your head from side to side. Be aware of how much more vivid everything around you now appears."

o

You'll now find that you are more aware of everything around you. You'll not only see more clearly but you'll also feel more a part of the world in which you live. Eyes really enjoy coming out of that frozen stance, and you'll find yours enthusiastic about their new freedom.

The minis in between the full sessions do not involve the exercises but will reinforce their effects. If your visual system starts to slide back into the old habits of tension, these minis will bring it right back into full, relaxed functioning. Use your rapid induction and then affirm the following:

o

"Eyes and visual system wonderfully relaxed. . . . My sight is effortless, spontaneous, and energetic. . . . My head and eyes move together as I edge and scan scenes for detail. I am interested in detail. . . . As I look into the distance, my oblique and ciliary muscles relax. . . . I breathe evenly and blink frequently as I see. . . . Movement is natural to my visual process. . . . I breathe and blink and keep my eyes moving. . . . My vision is much clearer than ever before. . . . I breathe, blink, move my eyes, and I see clearly."

WEEK SIX

Up to this point everything you have done has primarily been geared to relaxing your vision. Now your eyes will be able to maintain this relaxation while you engage them in some actual work. However, think of it more as play than as work, and your eyes will respond even more quickly. You will be stretching your vision out into the distance while you develop a skill known as *fusion*. Because of the space between them, each of your eyes sees a slightly different image. Fusion is the process of putting these two images together into one coherent clear one. Myopic eyes tend to focus in front of objects instead of directly on them, so this fusion exercise will also develop your ability to focus clearly on what you are looking at.

The exercise is called *string fusion*. You'll be sliding your gaze up and down a string containing a series of knots. Dr. Bates developed this exercise, but it is now widely used by optometrists who do visual training. However, they have found that the strain of forcing the eyes to focus together often causes astigmatism. This is because these doctors have not grasped the importance of relaxation in the visual process. The HypnoVision approach to string fusion surpasses even the standard Bates technique because of the deep relaxation maintained by doing the exercise while hypnotized.

For most of you, a six-foot length of string will be satisfactory for this exercise. You can use any string, but I recommend the bright yellow cord sold at hardware stores. The intensity of the color will help your vision stretch into the distance. Tie five knots in the string at one-foot intervals. It helps to fold the string in half and tie the middle knot first, so the rest are easier to space evenly. Making each knot a double one is a good idea, as this makes it easier to see. Painting each knot with red nail polish will also help. The higher your degree of myopia, the more you'll need the doubled and red knots. If you find that it is very easy for you to see the knots during the exercise, you can benefit from making the string longer and adding more knots. Conversely, if you have a great deal of difficulty stretching your vision all the way to the last knot, make the exercise easier by having ten knots tied at six-inch intervals along the six feet of string. This way you'll be asking your eyes to make smaller adjustments, and they will respond more quickly. Their confidence will grow if they experience success, and more success will soon follow.

Here is how string fusion works. Familiarize yourself with the process before you do it in the actual session. Tie one end of the

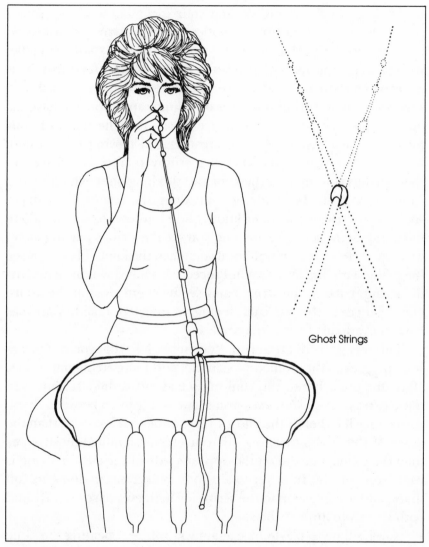

Ghost Strings

String Fusion

string to a doorknob or the back of a chair. Hold the other end against the end of your nose, and stand back until the string is taut between you and its anchor. Make sure your neck remains straight, as you'll create tension if it and your chin jut out. You can sit down to do the exercise, but be sure that the anchored end of the string is *lower* than the one at your nose.

Look down the string, letting your focus fall wherever seems comfortable. Close one eye and notice where the string is positioned in space. Now open that eye and close the other one. Notice that the string changes position. Go back and forth this way a few times. This is simply to show you that you see a different image with each eye. When you begin fusing your eyes on a single spot, you will have the optical illusion that two strings are crossing at the point of your focus. This exercise consists of creating and moving this illusion.

Focus your eyes on the knot closest to you. You should see two short strings coming into the knot and two long ones extending out from the knot in the shape of a V. Along the way on each string you'll be able to see the other knots. Slide your eyes slowly out along the string to the second knot, and you see the strings parting along with the focus of your vision until you reach the knot. There you see the strings crossing at the knot. Proceed this way down the length of the string, parting the strings and seeing them cross at the knots. Once you get to the last knot, seeing an inverted V, slide your eyes back in gradually to the first knot.

This was your first trial run. Remember it so that you can gauge your progress. If it seemed too simple, add more string and knots. If, on the other hand, you couldn't see as far as the last knot, add those extra ones so your eyes won't have so far to go between them. Also notice if either of the ghost strings appeared less clear than the other. If this is the case, one of your eyes is significantly stronger than the other. The eye on the opposite side of the clearer string is your stronger eye. In order to aid your weaker eye in doing its full share, add a suggestion to the script for both eyes to see clearly and both strings to appear the same.

Now it's time to play! Once again you will be repeating the same session twice a day. If your eyes should begin to feel strained during the eyes-open part of the session, close them and visualize doing the exercise until they have relaxed, then open them again and continue.

Have your string set up nearby, induce your hypnosis, and follow this script:

o

"Palm your eyes and let them relax into the darkness. Feel how well they have learned to let go and relax. . . . Deeply, wonderfully relaxed. . . . Your eye muscles are relaxed, aligned, and balanced. . . . Your eyes work as a perfectly coordinated team. They each see slightly different images, but your brain effortlessly fuses these two images into one clear one. The optic center of your brain directs your eyes to coordinate their focus perfectly, and it clearly interprets the images sent to it as one clear one. . . . Your eyes remain relaxed as they play with the string fusion exercise. . . . Your ciliary and oblique muscles relax as you stretch your vision into the distance, and you see clearly. . . . Imagine now that you are doing the string fusion exercise. See the string and the knots stretching from your nose to the anchor. Imagine focusing on the knot closest to you. Clearly see the short ghost strings coming into it and the long ones extending out from it in a V shape. You are also aware of the four knots along each of the ghost strings. Now imagine sliding your eyes out the string to the second knot, the strings parting as you move your focus out. At the second knot you see two strings coming back to you, a knot on each, and the other two extending into the distance, each containing three more knots. Imagine sliding your gaze on down to the third knot, strings parting, and seeing a perfect X at the knot. Every string coming out of the knot has two knots on it. In your imagination slide on to the fourth knot, strings parting. Long strings coming back toward you, three knots on each, shorter ones extending beyond, one knot on each. Now slide your vision down to the last knot, strings parting, two strings coming back at you from the knot, each with four knots evenly spaced along it. And now imagine sliding your gaze back to the first knot, seeing the strings part and then cross at each one of the knots. . . . Once you've imagined yourself back at the first knot, slide your way out again to the last one. See the process clearly. . . . Now allow the image to fade away. Your entire visual system understands how to fuse and stretch your vision in and out properly. You see clearly as you play with the fusion string. Your eye muscles are relaxed, aligned, and balanced, and you see clearly. Your ciliary and oblique muscles relax as you look down the string, and you see clearly. The optic center of your brain instructs your eyes to fuse and see clearly, and it interprets the images it receives as clear. Eyes relaxed and sight clear as you play with the fusion string. . . . In a few moments you will be opening your eyes and sitting or standing. You will be steady and perfectly balanced even though you will remain hypnotized. Remaining in a deeply relaxed hypnotic state, relax your hands down from your eyes. Swing or roll your head from side to side, and then gradually open your eyes, blinking softly, seeing clearly. . . . Position yourself with the fusion string suspended tightly between your nose and the anchor you have chosen for it. Focus your gaze on the knot closest to you. See the strings coming in and out of it. Be aware of the four knots on each string extending out into the distance in the shape of a V. Breathe, blink, and relax your neck and shoulders. Neck straight, chin pulled a little in. Take a deeper breath in, and as you let it out slide your focus down the string to the second knot, seeing the strings part as you move your eyes down to the knot. Breathe, blink, be aware of the string coming in, each having one knot, and the longer strings going into the distance, each with three knots. Take another deeper breath in, and let it out along with the sliding of your eyes to the third knot, observing the parting strings along the way. Breathe, blink, and be aware of the perfect X shape and the two knots on each string. Another deeper breath, and let it out along with your slide to the fourth knot, watching the strings part. Breathe, blink, and relax your neck and shoulders as you clearly see the longer strings coming back toward you, each with three knots, and the shorter strings extending into the distance, one knot on each. A deeper breath, and let it out as you slide to the last knot, strings parting, seeing strings in an inverted V shape coming back at you, four knots on each. Breathe, blink, relax. Eyes relaxed, balanced, aligned. Seeing clearly. . . . Now another deep breath, and let it out as you slide your gaze back in to the fourth knot. Breathe, blink, see clearly the knot where the strings cross, the single knots on each of the strings extending into the distance, the three knots on each string coming in to you. A deeper breath, let it out as you slide in to the third knot, seeing the perfect X, two knots on every string coming out of the knot. Breathing, blinking. . . . Exhaling as you slide in to the second knot, watching the strings part, observing the three knots on each string going into the distance and the single knots on the strings coming in to you. Breathing, blinking. Another deeper breath and an exhalation as you slide in to the first knot. Aware of the V-shaped strings extending into the distance, each having four knots. . . . Now at the same leisurely pace, accompanied by those exhalations as you slide, go through the same process again . . . gradually working your way out to the last knot. Your ciliary and oblique muscles relax as you stretch your vision into the distance. Neck and shoulders relaxed. Face and eyes relaxed. With every outward slide your fusion and clarity improve. . . . When you have reached the last knot, slide your way gradually back in to the first one. Breathing, blinking, relaxing. . . . Now speed up your sliding as you move to the end of the string and back again. Take in an especially deep breath, and exhale as you slide all the way to the last knot, watching the strings part, seeing them cross at each knot. Pause there and breathe and blink as you observe the clear knot and the strings with four knots extending back to you. Another deep breath, and let it out as you slide all the way back in. . . . Do this whole faster process once more. Breathing, blinking, relaxing. You see more clearly each time you do this exercise. Eyes relaxed, balanced, aligned. . . . Now slide out to the last knot one more time, slowly again this time, with an exhalation accompanying the slide to each knot. Blinking. Eyes, face, neck, and shoulders relaxing as you slide your vision into the distance. Seeing the string and knots clearly. . . . Now put the string down and return to palming your eyes. . . . Feel them totally relaxing into the soothing darkness. . . . In a

moment I'll count down from three to one. With each number feel yourself moving down, relaxing down. Three—every
muscle letting go as you sink into relaxation. Two—deeper
down, wonderfully relaxed. One—much deeper, totally relaxed. . . . During this rest period your eyes and visual system
are able to integrate fully the work you have just done. . . .
Every time you do the string fusion exercise, you see more
clearly. Your eye muscles are balanced, relaxed, aligned. Your
oblique and ciliary muscles relax when you look into the
distance. The optic center of your brain directs your eyes
to see clearly, and it fuses the images sent to it into one
clear image. . . . Seeing more clearly all the time. You are
ready for clear vision. You deserve clear vision. Your vision is
rapidly improving. . . . Wonderfully, deeply relaxed, inte-
grating your new visual skills. . . . It feels so good to improve
your vision. . . . Your vision is improving and you know it. . . .
Every time you do the string fusion exercise, your vision
improves. . . . Eyes relaxed, balanced, aligned. . . . Deeply relaxed. . . . In a few moments I'm going to begin counting
from one to five. With each number up you will become more
consciously alert while at the same time your subconscious
mind even more fully integrates the healing effects of the
string fusion work. . . . One—deepening your breathing,
coming up, confident of your ever-improving vision. Two—
feeling refreshed, your eyes relaxed and energized. Three—
halfway up, noticing the moist relaxation in your eyes. You
see more clearly than before. Four—almost all the way back.
Deeper breaths. Eyes relaxed, balanced, aligned, fusion ability improved. Come all the way back when you hear the next
number. Five—a deep breath and a stretch as you remove
your hands from your closed eyes. Alert and refreshed. Seeing better than ever. When you open your eyes, blink softly
and swing your head gently from side to side. You've done
good work, you see more clearly."

o

Your minisessions will keep reminding your eyes that they now work as a coordinated team and see more clearly than before. The minisessions don't involve the exercise itself, just the reminder that it is having a positive effect on your vision. After using your rapid induction, palm your eyes and affirm the following concepts to yourself:

o

"My eyes are relaxed, balanced, and aligned. . . . My eyes function as a relaxed, perfectly coordinated team. . . . My brain directs my eyes to work together and see clearly, and it fuses the images sent to it into single, clear images. . . . When I look into the distance, my ciliary and oblique muscles relax. . . . As I see I breathe and blink, and my shoulders, neck, head, face, and eyes remain relaxed. . . . My eyes are rounder, and shorter from front to back than before. I am ready for clear vision. I deserve clear vision. I am confident that my vision is improving. It all feels so very, very good."

o

During this week you'll notice how rapidly your eyes adapt to this exercise. Mastering the work involved will vastly increase their confidence as well as their skill. You'll feel this confidence spilling over into your general sense of well-being. You're making positive changes within yourself, and you'll enjoy that sense of accomplishment.

WEEK SEVEN

You're ready now to stretch your vision farther into the distance. At the same time, you will be increasing your eyes' ability to shift from close range into the distance. This is known as accommodation. It was happening while you were sliding your gaze out the fusion string, but now greater distance will be involved. Your ciliary muscles will learn to relax even more so that you will see more clearly in the distance.

For this exercise you'll be using the Near and Far letter charts that are supplied at the back of the book. They are identical except for size. Tear the page out or make a photocopy and cut apart the charts. Put the Far Chart, the big one, on a well-lighted wall at eye level. You can either sit or stand while you do the exercise. You'll be holding the small one, the Near Chart, in one hand at a comfortable reading distance. You want to be far enough away from the Far Chart so that the letters are just beginning to blur. This way your vision has room to improve during the session. If you mark each place where you sit or stand with a piece of tape, you'll have the positive reinforcement of seeing your progress as the pieces of tape get farther and farther away from the chart on the wall. As with the string fusion exercise, you'll be repeating the same one twice a day. You will also be visualizing doing the exercise effortlessly and clearly before you actually do it.

Have your charts ready, but first induce your hypnotic state and let the following soak into your subconscious:

o

"Palm your eyes and relax into the soothing darkness. Feel how quickly your eyes relax. Quickly and very deeply. Wonderfully relaxed. . . . Your oblique muscles completely relaxed. . . . Your ciliary muscles relaxed and energized, able to shift your lenses into the shape necessary for clear vision when you look into the distance. . . . Whenever you look into the distance, your ciliary muscles relax, your lenses spring into a convex shape, and you see clearly. . . . In a few moments you will visualize shifting your focus from near letters to distant ones. As you do this, your ciliary muscles and lenses will respond perfectly, just as if you were doing this exercise with your eyes open. The optic center of your brain will direct your ciliary muscles to perform optimally, and it will interpret the images sent to it as clear. . . . Now imagine you are standing back from a white piece of paper with the black letter *F* on it. But let the *F* appear a little blurry and a little gray instead of dark black. Now imagine looking at a white card in your hand and seeing an *F* on it. This one is very clear, and there is a sharp contrast between the white background and the dark, black *F*. Study the *F*, noting that it is made up of three black lines and that it stands out clearly against the white. As you do this the optic center of your brain is memorizing the *F*. In a moment it will direct your eyes to function so well that the distant *F* will seem just as clear as the close one. It does that now as you imagine looking out at the distant *F*. Now you see it clearly, clear black lines against the white background. Your brain directed your ciliary muscles to relax, they did, and the image became clear. Both your brain and eyes are capable of making these adjustments so you see clearly in the distance. . . . Now replace the *F* with an *O*, but let it seem farther away, so as the *F* was in the beginning, now the *O* is a little gray and blurry. Imagine looking at the white card in your hand and seeing a clear, black *O*. Study its shape and be aware of the contrast between the black and the white. Your brain is memorizing this *O* and will direct your eyes to see it clearly in the distance. Imagine looking up at the distant *O* and now seeing it perfectly clearly. Your eyes and brain are capable of making the necessary adjustments so you see clearly in the distance. Let the *O* fade away and replace it with an *E*, farther away now and just a little blurry and gray. Imagine looking down at the card in your hand and seeing a clear, black *E* against the white background. Study it, noticing the four black lines that make it up. Your brain is memorizing the *E* so it can instruct your eye muscles to relax when they look at the distant *E* and see it clearly. Imagine looking up now and seeing the far *E* just as clearly as the near one. Your eyes have adapted as they needed to so that you see clearly in the distance. One more letter now. Let the *E* fade away and replace it with *M*. This letter is farther away than the last and appears softer and grayer. Bring your mental vision down to the white card in your hand and see there a clear, black *M* in contrast to the white background. Study it, noting the four lines that make the *M*. Your brain is memorizing it so it can direct your eyes to adjust enough to see the distant *M* clearly. Imagine looking up and out now at the distant M, visualizing the letter M clearly now, black against white, all the lines distinct. Eyes and eye muscles relaxed, lenses convex. Good, your brain and eyes have learned how to adjust for clear distance vision. Soon they will practice this skill with your eyes open and will continue improving your distance vision. . . . First relax more deeply into the darkness. Eyes relaxed and energized. Ciliary and oblique muscle able to relax even more when you look into the distance. Brain able to direct the proper functioning of your eyes and able to interpret images sent to it clearly. . . . Wonderfully relaxed, ready to see clearly in the distance. . . . Even though you will still be hypnotized when you open your eyes, you will be alert and perfectly steady and balanced. Now, remaining in a re-laxed, hypnotic state, take your hands down from your eyes. Let them begin readjusting to the light behind your closed lids. Then swing your head gently from side to side as you open your eyes, blinking softly. . . . Position yourself for the accommodation exercise now, holding the small chart and being far enough way from the large one so that the letters are a little blurry and grayish. Look at the first letter on the near chart, the F. Blink and breathe as you edge around it. Notice the contrast between the black and the white. Close your eyes now and remember the F clearly, a vivid contrast between the white background and the three black lines that make up the F. Your brain remembers how this F looks and will direct your eyes to see it clearly in the distance. Your ciliary and oblique muscles will relax when you look at the distant F, and you will see it clearly. Take in a deep breath now, and as you let it out look at the F on the far chart. Eyes relaxing. Blink and breathe. See the three black lines making the F in contrast to the white background. Edge the distant F, tracing its three lines with your nose. See the F clearly. . . . Now look back down to the second letter on the near chart, the O. Study it, edge it, aware of the contrast between the black and the white. Close your eyes and clearly remember the O, black against the white background. . . . Take in a deep breath, let it out while blinking and shifting your focus to the distant *O*. Eyes relax, you see the *O* clearly, sharp contrast between the black *O* and the white background. Blink while you edge the *O*, and see it even more clearly. Neck and shoulders relaxed. . . . Look back down to the small card now, at the *E*. Blink, breathe, edge, and study it. Black against white. Close your eyes and remember the *E*, the four black lines that make it up against the white background. Your brain will direct your eyes to relax and adjust so you will see the *E* just as clearly in the distance. A deep breath in, let it out as you look at the distant *E*. See it clearly. Edge all its lines, see the contrast of black against white. Blink. . . . Look back down to the last letter in the first row of the small card, the *M*. Note the contrast and edge the *M*. Close your eyes and remember it. A breath in, and exhale as you open your eyes and see the distant *M* clearly. Make it even clearer by blinking and edging it. Ciliary muscles relaxed, eyes and lenses round. Seeing better all the time. . . . Look down to the first letter of the second row, the *B*. Blink while you edge it and note how black it is against the white background. Then close your eyes and remember the *B*. Your brain and eyes know how to make adjustments so you will see this *B* just as clearly in the distance. Take in your deep breath, blink as you let it out and look out to the far *B*. Eyes relaxed. Edge the *B*, noting its curves and straight line. It is very dark against the white background. . . . Look down to the second letter in the second row, the *J*. Study and edge it. Close your eyes and vividly remember it. Your eyes will relax when you look at it in the distance. Breathe in and exhale as you look down to the second letter in the second row, the *J*. Study and edge it, the straight line and the curved one. See the contrast of the white against the black. Close your eyes and vividly remember the *J*. Your brain knows how to direct your eyes to see the *J* clearly in the distance. Your eyes will relax when you look in the distance. Breathe in, and exhale as you open your eyes and look out at the distant *J*. Relaxing as you see. Brain interpreting the image clearly. Blink while you edge the *J*. Blinking and movement clear your vision. . . . Look back down to the third letter in the second row, the *K*. Edge it. See it as very black against the white. Close your eyes and visualize the *K*. See the three black lines that form it. Your eyes will relax as you look at it in the distance and you will see it clearly. Inhale, and exhale as you open your eyes and look out at the *K*. See the contrast of the black lines against the white background. Edge the *K*. Blinking. Your vision clearing even more. . . . Look back down to the last letter in the second row, the *P*. Edge it. See it as very black against the white background. Close your eyes and visualize the *P*. See the straight and curved lines that make it up. Your eyes will relax as you look at it in the distance and you will see it clearly. Inhale, exhale as you open your eyes, and look out at the distant *P*. See the contrast between the black and the white. Edge the *P*. Blinking and breathing. Your vision clearing even more. . . . Look down now to the first letter of the third row, the *A*. Shoulders and neck relaxed as you edge it. Close your eyes and remember the *A*. Three connected black lines against the white background. Inhale, and blink as you let the breath out and look out at the *A*. Eye muscles relaxing. Vision clearing. Edge the *A*. . . . Look down to the *C*. Edge its curve over and over. Eyes loose and relaxed. Close your eyes and visualize the *C*. Black on white. Your brain will direct your ciliary muscles to relax when you look at it in the distance. A breath in, exhale, and look out at the *C*. Ciliary muscles relax. Your brain interprets the *C* clearly. Blink and edge it. . . . Look back down to the *D*. Edge it and note the contrast of white and black. Shoulders relaxed. Close your eyes and visualize the *D* clearly. Your whole visual system will work in balanced harmony so you will see the *D* just as clearly in the distance. Breathe in, blink as you exhale, and look at the far *D*. Everything in your visual system relaxes and coordinates so you see the *D* clearly. Keep blinking as you edge it. . . . Look down now to the last letter in the third row, the *X*. Edge its crossed lines. Blinking. Relaxing. Close your eyes and remember the *X*. Black on white. You have the ability to see the *X* just as clearly in the distance. Inhale, then exhale as you look out to the *X*. Sharp, clear crossed black lines against the white background. Blink as you edge them. Movement clears your vision. . . . Look down to the first letter of the last row, the Q. As you edge it your brain memorizes it. Edge around in both directions. Close your eyes and remember the Q. See it clearly in your mind's eye. Black against white. Your brain will direct your eyes to see it just as clearly in the distance. A breath in, and let it out as you look at the far Q. Eyes relaxed. Blinking. Seeing the Q clearly as you edge it. . . . Look down to the next letter on the near chart, the R. As you edge it note the difference between the straight and curved lines. Blinking. Close your eyes and visualize the R clearly, very black against the white behind it. When you look at the far R, your ciliary and oblique muscles will relax, and you will see the R clearly. Inhale, and blink as you exhale and look out at the distant R. Eyes, neck, and shoulders relaxed. See clearly the contrast between the black R and the white background. Edge the R. . . . Look back down to the G. As you edge it your eyes are relaxed, balanced, and aligned. Close your eyes and remember the G clearly, black on a white background. Your eyes know exactly what to do to see it just as clearly in the distance. Breathe in, and exhale as you look out to the far G. It is clear and black against the white. Whole visual system relaxed and functioning beautifully. Blink as you edge the G. Blinking and movement clear your vision. . . . Look down at the last letter now, the S. Blink as you edge it. It is very black against the white. Close your eyes and clearly visualize the black S against the white background. You have skilled powers of accommodation, and when you look at the distant S you will see it clearly. A deep breath in, and blink as you let it out and look at the distant S. Ciliary muscles relaxed, perfect accommodation. Edge the S. You see it clearly, a black S against the white background. Eyes, neck, and shoulders relaxed. Vision clear. . . . Now do the chart accommodation once more, very quickly this time. Start with the F on the near chart. See it clearly and then immediately shift your eyes out to the distant F. Go on this way through the rest of the letters. . . . Breathe and blink as you shift your focus from the near letters to the far ones. . . . Ciliary muscles relax whenever you are looking at the distant letters. . . . Perfect accommodation. . . . Eyes relaxing when you look at the distant letters. . . . Eyes, neck, and shoulders relaxed. . . . Lenses shifting to change your focus. . . . You see just as clearly in the distance as at near-point. . . . Breathing and blinking. . . . Perfect accommodation. . . . Clear vision. . . . Clear vision. . . . When you have finished with the whole chart, make yourself comfortable for some palming. . . . Palm your eyes, and feel them let go into the soothing darkness. . . . Eyes strong and energized but wonderfully relaxed. . . . In a moment I'll count from three down to one. With each number down let yourself sink down into deeper and deeper relaxation. Three, moving down. Every muscle relaxing. Two, deeper down, deeper relaxed. When I count the last number, let your relaxation double with a wave of letting go and a pleasant, deep sinking sensation. One, doubling your relaxation. Completely relaxed. . . . Every time you practice the accommodation exercise, you see more clearly in the distance. Your eyes and brain understand how to shift your focus into the distance and see clearly. . . . You are ready for clear vision. You deserve clear vision. You see more clearly at all distances with each passing day. . . . Eyes wonderfully relaxed. . . . Whenever you look into the distance your ciliary muscles relax, your lenses become more convex, and you see clearly. . . . Everything in your visual system works in balanced harmony to bring you clear vision at all distances. . . . Everything in your visual system is relaxed, balanced, and aligned. . . . Your eyes are rounder, and shorter from front to back than before, and you see clearly. . . . Your eyes are alive with relaxation and vibrant energy. . . . In a few moments I'll count from one to five. At the subconscious level each number will reinforce all the positive benefits of this session. At the conscious level these numbers will bring you back to full waking alertness. One—coming up, relaxed and confident. Feeling really good. Two—breaths deepening, energy flowing. Your eyes feel rested yet vibrantly energetic. Three—halfway up. Notice how your eyes are moist with circulation and energy. Four—almost all the way back. So rested and refreshed. Feeling so good about your vision. Bring yourself all the way back to full conscious alertness when you hear the next number. Five—a deep breath and a stretch as you remove your hands from your closed eyes. Fully alert, wonderfully refreshed. Eyes relaxed and energized. When you open your eyes, swing your head gently from side to side and blink softly. Enjoy the freedom, power, energy, relaxation, and clarity of your vision."

o

Just as with the fusion string, you'll find your eyes adapting more and more to their new skills as the week goes on. You'll not only see more clearly in the distance, but you'll also experience an increasing freedom in your vision. It's as if your eyes have been released into a whole new world of color, detail, and activity. This is what healthy vision feels like. Isn't it wonderful?

Your minisessions will reinforce your accommodation skills and serve as reminders to practice them during the day by looking up frequently from close work. Use your rapid induction, palm your eyes, and repeat the following suggestions over and over:

o

"My eyes are wonderfully relaxed. . . . Relaxation is normal to them now. . . . They relax even more when I look into the distance. . . . I look into the distance frequently to relax my vision. . . . I see clearly in the distance as well as close up. . . . My brain instructs my ciliary and oblique muscles to relax when I look into the distance, and I see clearly. . . . My eyes are rounder than before, the perfect shape for clear vision at all distances. . . . I shift focus effortlessly from near to far, and I see clearly at all distances. . . . It feels so good to see so clearly."

o

WEEK EIGHT

Now we put it all together. Your eyes and visual system have been gradually incorporating all the suggestions and exercises. This week puts together everything you have learned in the last seven weeks. To be sure everything is fully covered, there will be two different full sessions. The first session will include string fusion, and the second contains the chart accommodation exercise, so set up your materials accordingly. The first session will also include sunning, so if you do it outside you may want to remain there for the fusion work.

Get into a comfortable position for palming, induce your hypnosis, and become fully immersed in the following script:

o

"Cup your palms over your closed eyes and feel them relax even more deeply. They are so good at relaxing. . . . Your ciliary and oblique muscles are relaxed, and your eyes are a nice round shape. . . . You are ready for clear sight, you deserve clear sight, and you enjoy seeing clearly at all distances. . . . The improvements you have achieved in your vision are lasting, and you will continue to improve your sight even more. . . . Circulation flows freely into your eyes, and they are relaxed and energized. . . . The optic center of your brain directs your eyes to see clearly, and it interprets images sent to it as clear. . . . In a few moments you will begin a massage that will further relax your eyes and send them even more circulation and energy. . . . Relax your hands down from your closed eyes, and come into a comfortable position for massaging. Let your head hang forward, stretch your arms up, then bend them at the elbows so that you can place your hands on your upper back on either side of your spine. Begin the stroking massage of your upper back and shoulders. With each stroke these muscles relax and circulation flows into your visual system. Your back and shoulders are able to maintain this relaxation. . . . Stroke your way up to your neck, and then shorten your strokes as you massage up your neck. Muscles relaxing, circulation flowing. It feels so good to relax, and your neck muscles will maintain this relaxation. . . . When you reach the base of your skull, spread your hands over the back of your head, and massage that bony ridge with your thumbs. Energy is released into your visual system as you massage. Massage out to the areas under your ears and then back to the center again. It feels so good. . . . Now dig your fingers into your scalp and give it a good loosening shake. Change the position of your fingers often so you free up your whole scalp. Feel the energy and circulation flowing into your scalp, into your eyes. Your back, shoulders, neck, and scalp wonderfully relaxed and energized. . . . Bring your massage down into your face. Loosen your forehead. Massage the hinges of your jaws and feel them let go. Then grasp your eyebrows and squeeze and massage them. Relaxation pouring in. This brief massage is just as effective as the longer ones. . . . Now massage the bony ridges surrounding your eyes. Feel the circulation and energy flowing into your eyes. Eyes expanding to a rounder, shorter shape as you massage. . . . Relax your hands down now and experience the wonderful glow of relaxation, circulation, and energy in your back, shoulders, neck, head, face, and eyes. . . . Your vision is healed and clear. . . . Palm your eyes again, and feel them sink into even deeper relaxation. . . . The positive effects of your massage are permanent. . . . Let your breath seem to flow into your eyes, feeling them expand slightly with your inhalations and let go completely with each exhalation. . . . Relaxing into the round shape necessary for clear vision. . . . Permanent relaxation in your ciliary and oblique muscles. . . . In a few moments you'll begin sunning and swinging, and their healing benefits will be even more profound than ever before. . . . Leaving your eyes *closed,* take your hands down and face the sun or a bright light you can imagine to be the sun. Feel the sun's soothing warmth penetrating your closed lids. Feel your face and eyes relaxing even more. . . . Now begin swinging your head from right to left across the sun. Observe that the sun seems to move in the

opposite direction of your swing. Your eyes enjoy this movement and relax even more. They relax and vibrate with life
and energy. Loose and energetic. . . . Change the direction of
your swing now so that you are moving your head up and
down across the sun. Breathe in its warmth and energy.
Shoulders and neck relaxing. Feel the massage to the optic
center of your brain. Eyes relaxed and energetic. . . . Begin
making large, looping circles around the sun now. Neck
relaxing even more. Eye muscles balancing and aligning.
Eyes floating along with the motion of your head. Relaxation
a permanent part of your visual system. . . . Reverse the direction of your circles. Breathe as you make loose, easy circles
around the sun. So relaxed, so free. Movement is a natural
part of your visual process. Eyes vibrating with energy, able
to see clearly. . . . Let go of the movement and palm your eyes.
Feel them relax into the soothing darkness. So relaxed and
yet so vibrantly alive. Muscles relaxed, balanced, aligned, and
eyes expanded and round. Vision healed and clear. . . . Keep
your eyes closed as you take down your hands. Imagine a
white three-by-five card suspended in the distance in front of
you. Give it a vertical black line in the center and a black dot
on either side of the line. Point your nose at the dot on the
right, then swing over to the one on the left. Swing back and
forth from dot to dot, observing that the line moves in the
opposite direction of your swing. Such a small movement and
yet it so completely relaxes your eyes. Movement is natural to
your sight. The black and white are in sharp contrast. . . . Let
go of the image on the card and replace it with a horizontal
black line across the center and a black dot above and below
the line. Point your nose at the top dot, then move it down to
the bottom one. Swing up and down across the black line
from dot to dot, enjoying the black line moving in the opposite direction of your swing. Eyes loose, energetic, balanced,
and aligned. Neck and shoulders relaxed, optic center of
your brain massaged. You see clearly. . . . Let go of the movement and the image, and feel the relaxation and the energy.
Palm your eyes again. Feel them relax even more. In a mo-

ment I'll count from three down to one. With each number down let your mental and physical relaxation deepen. Three, a pleasant sinking sensation. So relaxed. Two, deeper down, so very relaxed. One, way down. Completely relaxed. Your eyes, visual system, and subconscious mind fully accept all the positive benefits of the HypnoVision program. Relaxation, movement, and clarity are natural parts of your visual process. . . . In a few moments you will stand up for long swings. During them your eyes will relax and regain their natural balance and movement even more. You will be alert, yet still hypnotized and open to positive suggestions. Uncover your eyes now. Swing your head gently from side to side. Blink softly as you open your eyes. Find a place facing away from the sun for long swings. . . . With your feet shoulder width apart, begin swinging from side to side. Arms loose, eyes moving along with your head and body. Blink and breathe as you swing. Let the world slide by in the opposite direction of your swing. Clear details pop out at you as you swing by them. Your lenses and ciliary muscles are relaxed as you swing, and you see the world clearly as you let it slide by. Your eyes vibrate with movement and energy. It feels so good to relax and see clearly. These swings permanently restore freedom of movement to your eyes. Breathing and blinking are effortless, natural parts of your visual process. Energy flowing up your spine and into your visual system. Colors are bright and vividly clear. Vision so relaxed and clear as you swing. . . . Let go of the swinging now. Notice how good your eyes feel and how clearly you see. Take up your fusion string now, your back to the sun if you are outside. Look at the knot closest to your nose. Be aware of the two ghost strings extending out into the distance, each with four knots. Inhale, and let the breath out as you slide your gaze out the string to the second knot, watching the strings part. As you focus on the second knot, you are also aware of the ghost strings and their three knots. Your eyes work together in balanced harmony. Another breath in, and let it out as you slide out to the third knot. See the perfect X and be aware of the two knots on each ghost string. Your ciliary muscles relax as you stretch your vision into the distance. A deep inhalation. Blink as you let your breath out and slide to the fourth knot. The strings part so easily, and you see the fourth knot clearly. Be aware of the ghost strings and knots. Neck and shoulders relaxed. Another deep inhalation. Blink as you let it out and slide all the way out to the last knot. Ciliary muscles relaxing as you slide into the distance. The last knot is very clear, and the ghost strings coming in toward you each have four knots. Everything in your visual system relaxed and working as a coordinated team so that you see clearly. Now take in an especially deep breath, let it out slowly, blinking, and slide your eyes in one long smooth movement all the way back to the first knot. . . . Good. Take in another especially deep breath, and as you let it out slide all the way out to the last knot. Blink. Everything in your visual system relaxing and cooperating to make this an easy, smooth, clear slide. Seeing so very clearly. As your eyes focus in clear, balanced alignment on the last knot, you are also aware of the ghost strings with the four knots. . . . Put down your fusion string now, and make yourself comfortable for palming. . . . As you cup your hands over your closed eyes, relaxation instantly spreads throughout every muscle, cell, nerve, and fiber of your mind and body. In a moment I'll count down from five to one. Feel a pleasant downward sensation with each number down. By the number one you'll be completely relaxed. Five—letting go, sinking down. Four—every muscle relaxing. Eyes feeling so good. Three—deeper and deeper down. It feels so good to relax so completely. Two—even deeper. Feeling peaceful and quiet. When you hear the last number, let your relaxation double. One—all the way down, doubling your relaxation. Luxuriate in this total relaxation. . . . Your eyes are healed and your vision clear. Your eyes are shorter and rounder than before. Your oblique muscles are relaxed. Your ciliary muscles relax whenever you look into the distance, and you see clearly. Your eyes fuse and accommodate with clear, balanced precision. The optic center of your brain directs your eyes to see clearly, and it clearly interprets the images sent to it. Your whole visual system works perfectly, and you see clearly at all distances. You are ready for clear sight. You see clearly. It feels so good to see clearly. Movement and vibration are natural and effortless for your eyes, and you see clearly. It feels so good to see so clearly. . . . In a few moments I'll count from one to five. With each number up your subconscious mind will even more fully accept and integrate the positive effects of every exercise and suggestion. These numbers will also serve as reminders to your conscious mind that it is time to return to full alertness. One—your breath beginning to deepen. Feeling so good about the clarity of your vision. Two—coming up. Wonderfully relaxed and refreshed. Knowing you see clearly. Three—halfway up. Your eyes are moist with relaxation, circulation, and energy. You see clearly. Four—almost all the way up to full alertness. So confident of your clear vision. When you hear the last number come all the way back to conscious alertness. Feeling terrific. Five, all the way up. You see clearly. Take that deep breath, remove your hands from your closed eyes, and stretch and yawn. Swing your head gently from side to side and blink softly as you open your eyes. Enjoy the clarity of your vision."

o

Your other full session will incorporate the rest of the elements of the whole program. In the meantime, your minis will reinforce all the important visual concepts so that your subconscious will understand that now is the time for complete recovery of your clear vision. After your rapid induction, palm your eyes and affirm the following:

o

"My vision is relaxed, spontaneous, and clear. . . . I see clearly at all distances. . . . The farther I look into the distance, the more my ciliary and oblique muscles relax, and I see clearly. . . . As my ciliary muscles relax my lenses spring into the convex shape for distance vision and focus the images directly on my retina, and I see clearly. . . . The optic center of my brain directs my eyes to see clearly, and it interprets the images sent to it as clear. . . . I enjoy seeing clearly and I am interested in the details around me. . . . My eyes function in perfect relaxed alignment and I see clearly. . . . My shoulders, neck, face, and eyes are relaxed. They relax even more when I look into the distance, and I see clearly. . . . My breathing is even and I blink gently and frequently. . . . I edge and scan scenes for detail, and movement is natural to my vision. . . . I am absolutely confident of the clarity of my vision. . . . I see clearly."

o

Now let's top everything off with your final full session. Even though you go over all the elements rather quickly in both these sessions, your visual system is well primed to react to them quickly and fully. Reviewing the whole range of skills that you have built into your vision reminds it just how competent it is to see clearly.

Induce your hypnotic state of mind, and continue on with the following script:

o

"Palm your eyes, and immediately feel them relax even more. Your eyes understand how to relax now, and it is their natural state. Your vision is free, spontaneous, and relaxed. You see clearly at all distances. Everything in your visual system works in balanced harmony to bring you clear vision. During this session the suggestions for clear vision will be even more fully accepted by your subconscious and even more fully integrated into your visual system. In a few moments you will begin the acupressure massage. Its positive benefits will be more fully integrated into your visual system than ever before. You will remain in a pleasant deep state of hypnosis while you give yourself the acupressure massage. Bring your hands down from your closed eyes to the first acupressure points. Press and massage in firm circular movements with your thumbs on the indentations above the inside corners of your eyes. Breathe into this massage. You are releasing healing energy into your eyes and visual system. Vision healing, clear sight is yours once again. It feels so good. . . . Move on to the second points, using the thumb and index finger of one hand to massage gently the gristly spots in from the corners of your eyes. Releasing healing energy. Your eyes wonderfully relaxed and energized. It feels so good, and it is so heal-ing. . . . Move on to the third points now, the ones on your cheekbones a finger's width away from the edge of your nose. Press into them with your index fingers, and massage in circular motions. The energy is released and is healing your vision. You can feel it happening. It feels so very, very good. The healing you began so many weeks ago is now being completed. Breathe into the massage. Feel the healing en-ergy flow. . . . Move on to the last series of points, the ones on the bony ridges surrounding your eyes. Bend your index fingers and stroke with the knuckles from the inside corners of your eyes to the outer corners. First the top ridges and then the bottom ones. Top and bottom. Healing energy being released from all those acupressure points. You can feel it flowing into your eyes and visual system. It feels so good to heal your vision. You know you see clearly now. . . . Let go of the massage and palm your eyes again. As they relax even more deeply, you feel the healing effects of the acupressure massage. Your eyes are alive with balanced energy, and you see clearly. . . . Feel your breath going directly into your eyes. They are so relaxed and energized that they easily expand with each breath in and relax even more deeply with each breath out. . . . Expanding and relaxing into a shorter and rounder shape than before. . . . Now visualize your eyes. Your eyeballs, oblique extraocular muscles, ciliary muscles, and lenses. Imagine healing hands coming in to this picture. See and feel them begin to massage your oblique muscles. Imme-diately you experience deeper release and relaxation in these muscles. It feels so good as they let go. As they relax, you see and feel your eyeballs expanding into a rounder shape, shorter from front to back than before. . . . Now the hands move on to your ciliary muscles. The massage feels so good, and your ciliary muscles respond by loosening and relaxing.

As they do you can see and feel your lenses relax into a rounder, more convex shape. The shape necessary for clear distance vision. You see clearly in the distance. . . . Let the healing hands fade out of the picture, but maintain an image of your eyes. Add the rest of your visual system to it. Be aware of your retina, your optic nerves, the visual center of your brain. Feel that you are breathing into your eyes again, and this time you breathe in the golden light of healing energy. It fills your eyes, energizing and enlivening them. It travels down your optic nerves to the optic center of your brain. Everything alive and glowing with healing golden energy. You can feel it as well as see it. Pulsating with golden energy. Your eyes and vision healing. You see it, feel it, and know it. . . . Let the image fade and feel the positive healing benefits of the healing energy. Eyes feeling so good, you know you see clearly. . . . In a few moments you will open your eyes and edge and scan the scene around you for details. As you do your eyes will feel alive with movement and energy, and you will see the scene clearly. Relax your hands down now. Let your eyes begin their adjustment to the light under closed lids as you swing your head gently from side to side. When you open your eyes blink softly. . . . Following your nose, edge around the biggest shapes in your view. Breathing, blinking, and movement are natural to your visual process. The more you breathe, blink, and move your eyes, the clearer you see. After edging around objects, scan over them for more details. Your retinas are recording bits of visual information and sending them to the optic center of your brain. Your brain interprets what you see as clear. Everything working in perfect coordination, seeing clearly. Shoulders, neck, face, and eyes relaxed. Breathing and blinking. You enjoy picking out details. . . . Close your eyes for a moment and remember what you have seen. The details are vivid. . . . Open your eyes, and observe that anything you missed seems to jump out at you. Edge and scan these new details. Leading with your nose. Easy relaxed movements. . . . Close your eyes again and remember what you have seen. . . . Open your eyes, blinking softly, and observe the scene again. Now begin swinging your head and eyes from side to side across the view, and be aware of the color blue. All the blues jump out at you as you swing across the scene. Be aware of the color green as you swing. All the greens jump out at you. Seeing clearly as you swing. Now pick out a color of your own to be aware of as you swing, one you know occurs often in the scene in front of you. Observe how this color jumps out at you as you swing. Eyes so relaxed, energetic, and observant. . . . Let go of the swinging now, and position yourself so that you are ready to work with the accommodation charts, standing far enough away from the large chart so it is just a bit blurry. As you work with it your vision will adapt and improve and you will quickly see this chart clearly. Look at the *F* on the small chart in your hand. Blink while you edge and memorize it. Close your eyes and remember the *F*. Visualize it clearly and be aware of the contrast between the black and the white. When you look at the *F* in the distance, your ciliary muscles will relax and you will see it clearly. Breathe in and exhale as you look out to the distant *F*. Eyes adapting, seeing the *F* clearly. Blink as you edge it and observe it becoming ever more clear. Look down to the *O* on the near chart. Edge and memorize it. Close your eyes and remember it vividly. When you look out to the far *O*, your eyes will make the proper adjustment and you will see the *O* clearly. Inhale, exhale, and blink as you look at the distant *O*, seeing it clearly. Edge it, the movement further clearing your vision. Look in to the *E* on the small chart. Blink as you edge it. Close your eyes and remember it clearly, black on white. You will see it just as clearly when you look to the far chart. Breathe in, let the breath out as you open your eyes and focus clearly on the far *E*. Your vision is so adaptable and you see so clearly. Edge the *E*, movement makes it even more clear. Now look down to the last letter in the first row, the *M*. Edge and memorize it. Close your eyes and clearly remember the *M*, black on a white background. The optic center of your brain will direct your eyes to see the *M* clearly in the distance. Inhale, let the breath out, and look to the

distant *M*. Ciliary muscles relax, you see the *M* clearly. You
see the sharp contrast between the black *M* and the white
background even more vividly as you blink and edge the
M. . . . Put down your near chart now and return to palming
your eyes. . . . In a moment I'll begin counting down from
five to one. With each number down experience a pleasant
downward sensation and deepen your relaxation. Five—
everything letting go as you move downward. Eyes relaxing
totally. Four—deeper down, feeling lazy and comfortable.
Three—every muscle, nerve, and cell completely relaxing.
Two—deeper into pleasant hypnotic relaxation. When you
hear the next number, let your relaxation double. One—way
down, doubling your relaxation. So wonderfully peaceful
and relaxed. So completely confident of your clear vision.
Everything in your visual system has learned to relax and
adapt so that you see clearly. . . . Your ciliary and oblique
muscles function in a state of dynamic relaxation. They relax
even more when you look into the distance, and you see
clearly. . . . The optic center of your brain directs the rest of
your visual system to function optimally. Your brain interprets the images sent to it as clear. . . . Your vision is alive with
energy and movement, and you see clearly. Breathing and
blinking are integral parts of your visual functioning, and
you see clearly. . . . Through the power of your subconscious
mind, you have healed and cleared your vision. . . . In a few
moments I'll count from one to five. While your conscious
alertness is reactivated by these numbers, your subconscious
mind will more deeply accept the clarity of your vision. By the
number five you'll be fully alert, seeing clearly. One—deepen
your breathing. Coming up. Totally confident of your clear
vision. Two—energy flowing, feeling refreshed, and knowing
your vision is clear. Three—halfway up. Feel the circulation,
relaxation, and energy in your eyes. You see clearly. Four—
almost all the way up. Energy flowing. Knowing you see
clearly. When you hear the next number, you'll be fully alert,
feeling wonderful, absolutely certain of the clarity of your
vision. Five—Fully alert. Refreshed and relaxed. Feeling so

good about the clarity of your vision. Take your hands down from your closed eyes as you stretch and yawn. When you open your eyes, swing your head from side to side, blink softly, and see clearly."

o

Congratulations! By now you should have regained much, if not all, of your visual clarity. No doubt you'll also feel that your whole outlook on life has expanded as well. You are a powerful person who has achieved wonderful positive changes within yourself. Let this be just the beginning for you. It is the birthright of every one of us to grow continually and fulfill our potentials. You have regained your physical visual potential. Carry on in the same spirit and turn all your visions into reality!

To maintain your improved visual acuity, you can simply give yourself a few minisessions every week or so. You might also want occasionally to indulge yourself in one of your favorite full-length sessions every now and then. The massages and the swings are the usual choices. I must admit that some people do just fine without any maintenance program, but I encourage these reminders to your visual system.

If You Haven't Improved Your Sight as Much as You Desired

If you want more visual improvement than you've experienced so far, it's time to get out your pendulum. Most of you won't need to go beyond the first few questions. If you've been myopic for a good many years, chances are this eight-week session just wasn't long enough to undo all those negative habits and programs. Your subconscious will tell you if you need more work, and you will even be able to pinpoint the areas needing the most work. Some of you, on the other hand, may now determine that there are some emotional factors that need to be dealt with before your vision can come up to par. If this is the case, you'll move to Chapter 12, on "Regression."

Establish your yes, no, I-don't-know, and I'm-not-ready-to-talk-about-it responses with your pendulum. Once you've done this, go on and ask your subconscious the following questions:

1. In order to see clearly, do I need to spend more time working with the HypnoVision program?
2. Do I need more work with the entire program? If you receive a no answer to this question, ask your subconscious about each element of the program, using the following questions:
    a. Do I need to strengthen my belief in the ability of my vision to improve?
    b. Do my ciliary muscles need to relax more for distance vision?
    c. Do my oblique extraocular muscles need to relax more?
    d. Do my eyeballs need to be shorter and rounder?
    e. Do I need more movement in my vision?
    f. Do I need to blink more frequently?
    g. Do I need more massages?
    h. Will improving my posture help my vision? If you get a yes answer to this, it's time for an exercise or body therapy program!
    i. Do I need to improve my ability to visualize?
    j. Do I need more fusion work?
    k. Do I need more accommodation work?

Based on the answers you come up with to these questions, you can go back through the program and tailor-make your own sessions. If you think there's still more involved, go on with the following questions:

3. Am I emotionally ready to see clearly?
4. Do I want to see more clearly? This is an interesting question. It is different from not being ready yet. Some people find that they really like their vision the way it is.
5. Is it okay to explore the emotions and events that caused the blurring of my vision?

Do what you need to do, what you're ready to do, and continue on with your progress!

7

The Presbyopia Program

Sometime after the age of forty most people begin to notice a peculiar change in their bodies—their arms become shorter and shorter until they are unable to hold a book far enough away to see the print clearly. Oh, I know, it's a silly joke, but if you wear reading glasses you know exactly what I mean. The good news is that you don't have to submit to the ravages of time on your vision any more than on the rest of your body and your mind. When your spine begins to stiffen with age you can either grab a cane or you can respond with a positive attitude and a good program of exercise and nutrition. It's the same with your eyes. You already have the right attitude or you wouldn't be reading this book. Good for you!

The best news is that presbyopia responds beautifully to the HypnoVision approach. Beautifully and quickly. This program takes only four weeks. In fact, if you haven't needed reading glasses for too long, your eyes may regain their nearpoint clarity even more quickly. However, even if this is the case, I still recommend that you complete the entire program. You want to be sure that your eyes and subconscious have fully integrated this method for maintaining as well as regaining your near vision.

Alicia, a feisty senior citizen who hadn't needed reading glasses until she was over sixty, was a client of mine who illustrated this need to stay with the program for a while. Because she was physically active and had needed the glasses only for a short time, she responded so well that she could read fine print after her second session. Being a free spirit who didn't take well to regimes, she stopped even her home minisessions. After two weeks her near vision began to blur again. I worked with her twice more and made her promise to keep up a maintenance program. That was three years ago, and her Christmas cards to me proclaim happily that her eyes and mind are remaining "as young and impudent as ever!"

As you'll remember from Chapter 3, presbyopia occurs when the lenses of your eyes lose their flexibility. This is due primarily to a lack of circulation within the lenses and is accentuated by a loss of tone in the muscles controlling their shape. This is a natural consequence of aging, but it can be compensated for by nutrition, exercise, relaxation, and attitude, just like all the other physical problems associated with aging. I have to admit that during my early days of vision work I was rather surprised by how quickly presbyopes regained their nearpoint acuity. I was much younger then, and my consciousness was raised by these people who refused to give up their youthful flexibility. As I write this book I am forty-four and have an even deeper appreciation for all the good things that come with age. And I also now have this improved method of reversing presbyopia or keeping it at bay, so that I can maintain my own close vision while I am able to help others.

Before we get into the program itself, there are some life-style pointers that can help you make even more rapid progress. The foremost is that old nemesis, cigarette smoking. How many reasons do you need to give it up? Smokers become presbyopic nearly ten years earlier than nonsmokers. Remember that your lenses are made up of layers of tissue that receive their nutrients through very finely filtered circulation. Smoking is devastating to your circulation. When it is impaired your eyes suffer immediately. Without circulation your lenses become dry and inflexible and can no longer shift into the shape for close vision. You can compensate somewhat with increased exercise, an improved diet, and antioxidant vitamins, but getting rid of the cigarettes will help a lot more.

Any form of exercise that promotes good circulation will benefit your vision at all distances, but especially at the nearpoint. I'm in favor of moderate exercise programs and particularly fond of brisk walking. But at the very top of my list is yoga. It's easily learned, adaptable to any fitness level, and can't be beat for increasing circulation to all your internal organs, including your eyes. I've been teaching yoga even longer than I have been teaching vision improvement techniques, and it's been a constant joy to watch people becoming more youthful and vital with each passing week. But, whatever form of it you choose, exercise keeps you young, and that's certainly what reversing presbyopia is all about.

Lightening up on your diet will also increase your circulation and youthfulness. I don't necessarily mean eating less, but do look at the quality of what you are consuming. All those nasties you already know about, such as cholesterol, sugar, and white flour, are going to impact your sight as well as your general health. As we get older it becomes even more difficult for our bodies to handle impurities. Questioning the subconscious of one client, for example, revealed that consumption of fast-food hamburgers was the culprit behind the lack of circulation into his eyes. So load up on those vegetables, fruits, and complex carbohydrates. And, yes, carrots really are good for your eyesight, especially your night vision.

Along with what you eat, consider what you drink. Caffeine and alcohol actually dehydrate you, cutting down both nutrients and circulation into your eyes. I can't overemphasize the importance of plenty of good, clean water in your diet. I've sometimes had to use hypnotic suggestion to get clients started on water, but once they experience the difference it makes they need no further urging. Try it with a slice of lemon. You'll like it!

Now, with your life-style contributing to your better eyesight, let's move on to the HypnoVision program itself. It consists of five sessions a day. Two are full ones, which average about twenty minutes each, and the other three are minisessions, which take only three to five minutes apiece. If you absolutely don't have the time for both the long sessions, do what you can and make your "week" a little longer. However, hypnotic relaxations, regardless of the subject addressed, are so rejuvenating that you'll find you have more energy than ever before, so I strongly urge you to make the necessary time. You will remain hypnotized for the entirety of each session, even when it includes exercises as well as suggestions. If you've ever seen a hypnosis stage show you realize that physical activity and even speech are quite possible during the trance. It feels more like being awake, but you'll still be in that altered state of consciousness that produces the changes we are after.

WEEK ONE

There are no exercises this first week, just powerful hypnotic suggestions. The object is to open circulation into your lenses and to attain an absolute conviction within your subconscious that positive changes are taking place. Your circulation is controlled by your subconscious mind, and it responds almost immediately to suggestions. In my everyday hypnotherapy practice I often work with circulatory problems accompanying far more serious health problems than visual defects, and they too respond beautifully to suggestions for improvement. Don't be surprised if you begin to see more clearly at nearpoint during this first week.

You will be using the same script for both full sessions this first week, whereas the following weeks will utilize a different script for each. The short script for the minisessions will be the same for the entire program. If you become truly proficient at inducing a deep state of hypnosis through the rapid-induction technique, you can use it to begin your full sessions as well. However, I urge you to use the full-length induction whenever you have the time, since many people never reach the same depth with the rapid induction as they do the full one. Entering into a deep hypnotic state is crucial to the success of the program.

Once you have induced your hypnosis, you will be covering your closed eyes with the palms of your hands during the suggestion segment. Palming is wonderfully relaxing to the eyes, and the electrical energy that is emitted through the palms of your hands stimulates circulation in your eyes. Don't actually touch your eyelids with your palms, but rather cup them over your eyes, applying gentle pressure to the bony ridges under your eyebrows and above your cheekbones so that your eyes feel like they are floating in between. (See illustration on page 58.) If you do the session sitting up, you can simply rest your elbows on a table. If you prefer to lie down, you can put pillows under your arms for support or give yourself some added suggestions for the lightness and comfort of your arms.

Now you're ready. This script begins where the induction (see page 46) leaves off.

o

"Cup your palms over your closed eyes and feel them relax into the soothing darkness. . . . As you relax into the darkness, feel it taking you even deeper into hypnotic relaxation. . . . More relaxed with each easy breath out. . . . In this state of deep relaxation your eyes are completely at rest, completely relaxed, completely open to positive suggestions. . . . This total relaxation increases the healthy flow of circulation throughout your entire body and especially into your eyes. . . . The circulation into your eyes is increasing right now. . . . Healthy open circulation into every nerve, muscle, cell, and fiber of your eyes. . . . Every nerve, muscle, cell, and fiber of your entire visual system is flooded with healthy circulation. . . . Nourishing, rejuvenating circulation is flowing into every part of your eyes, and especially into the lenses of your eyes. . . . An open healthy flow of circulation is rejuvenating the lenses of your eyes. . . . Vital nutrients are flowing unimpeded into the lenses of your eyes. . . . Through this flow of circulation and nutrients your lenses are regaining their youthful moisture and elasticity. . . . Your lenses are absolutely capable of regaining their youthful elasticity and moisture. . . . You are completely confident of your own ability to increase circulation into your eyes through tapping into the power of your subconscious mind, the control tower of your physiological functioning. . . . Your subconscious now sends nourishing circulation into the lenses of your eyes. . . . Your lenses respond to this increased circulation by becoming moist and flexible. . . . Your lenses are regaining their youthful flexibility and their ability to focus clearly at close range. . . . You are young in spirit, flexible, and adaptable, and your eyes follow suit. . . . You and your vision are flexible. . . . Your mind is powerful and clear, and so is your vision. . . . The lenses of your eyes are healthy, moist, and flexible. . . . The circulation into the lenses of your eyes improves with each passing day. . . . You desire to see clearly up close, so your subconscious mind directs the flow of circulation into your eyes to increase. It is completely within the power of your subconscious to increase the flow of circulation into the lenses of your eyes. . . . Healthy rejuvenating circulation is flowing into your eyes. . . . Your vision is rejuvenating. . . . Your vision is rejuvenating. . . . The dead cells in the lenses of your eyes are washed away by the circulation flowing into them and are replaced by new, healthy cells. . . . Your vision is youthful, vibrant, and flexible. . . . Your lenses are so moist and flexible that they can adjust effortlessly so you see clearly up close as well as in the distance. . . . The ciliary muscles that control the shape of your lenses are youthful, fit, and toned. . . . Your ciliary muscles easily adjust your moist, flexible lenses into the flatter, more concave shape necessary for close work, and you see clearly up close. . . . With every passing day, with every positive suggestion and every vision exercise you practice, your nearpoint vision improves. You are absolutely certain that you are regaining your clear near vision. . . . Your entire visual system now performs optimally. . . . The optic center of your brain gives clear specific instructions to your ciliary muscles and lenses so that they adjust fully for near as well as distance vision, and you see clearly at all distances. You see clearly up close. . . . Your lenses are flushed with circulation. Your lenses are moist, nourished, and flexible, and you see clearly up close. . . . Your mind is youthful and flexible, and so is your vision. . . . It feels so good to regain the youthful flexibility of your vision. You feel relaxed, vibrant, and rejuvenated, and so do your eyes. . . . You know your near vision is improving. . . . In a few

moments I'll begin counting from one to five. At the subconscious level these numbers will allow your mind and eyes
to accept and integrate even more fully every positive suggestion that has been made. At the conscious level these
numbers will serve as signals that it is time to return to full
alertness. By the number five you'll be wide awake, alert, refreshed, and fully confident of your increasing ability to see
clearly up close. . . . One—coming up. Increase your energy
by deepening your breathing. Two—more alert, energy flowing. Feeling so relaxed and refreshed. Three—halfway up.
Be aware of your eyes and feel the moisture and circulation
within them. Four—almost all the way back. So rested, refreshed, and confident of your improving vision. When you
hear the next number, bring yourself all the way back to full
conscious alertness. Five—all the way back now. Wonderfully
refreshed, relaxed, and energized. Positively rejuvenated.
Remove your hands from your closed eyes and indulge in a
nice stretch and a yawn. Let your eyes begin readjusting to
the light under your closed lids. Then, when you open them,
blink softly while you gently swing your head from side to
side. Enjoy the freedom and clarity in your vision."

o

It's usually temporary, but many presbyopes can see printed pages
clearly after their very first session. Even though it doesn't usually
last too long, it demonstrates the regenerative power of the eyes. On
the other hand, if your eyes don't respond immediately, just give
them a little more time. I have yet to see the massages you'll experience in the second session fail to bring about dramatically increased
clarity of vision. Meanwhile, the sessions this week will ready your
eyes for more change. And the minisessions in between will keep
your subconscious reminded that positive changes are taking place.

Three minutes is plenty of time for the minisessions, including
the rapid induction and the awakening procedure. But, of course, if
you can stretch them out to five minutes, so much the better. The
refreshing quality of these minis will be reflected in your general
attitude and energy level as well as in your vision. You can easily

commit the concepts to memory, as the exact phrasing and order is not as important as in the full sessions. However, if you find you have trouble concentrating during the sessions, you can tape them. A few of my clients take tape recorders to work and find a private place to spend a few minutes with taped minisessions. If you do this, be sure to change the pronoun back into the third person, from "I" to "you."

Use your rapid induction (see page 50). Then, palming your eyes, think the following suggestions over and over to yourself:

o

"My eyes are relaxed and circulation flows freely into them. . . . Circulation flows freely into the lenses of my eyes. . . . My lenses receive healthy nutrients through the free flow of circulation into them. . . . My lenses are moist and flexible. They easily shift focus so I see clearly at near-point. . . . I am youthful and flexible and so are the lenses of my eyes. . . . My lenses are flexible and my ciliary muscles are elastic and fit. My ciliary muscles effortlessly shift my lenses so I focus clearly up close. . . . I am absolutely confident that my vision is rejuvenating. . . . My eyes, my mind, and my body are relaxed, flexible, energetic, and vibrantly alive."

o

After you count yourself up you and your vision will be wonderfully refreshed. Throughout the week you'll find that your vision and your skill as a hypnotic subject will steadily increase. They are both, after all, learned skills. By the end of this week your vision will be ready to respond to the healing power of massage.

WEEK TWO

This week your full sessions will combine massage with hypnotic suggestions. Each session is composed of a different massage. During the first you will work your way systematically up from your shoulders and neck, over your head, into your face, and around your eyes. These areas are all interconnected with your visual system, so the effects will reach deeply into your eyes as well as the actual areas you massage. During the second session you will be using a Chinese acupressure massage that will stimulate the flow of energy into your entire visual system.

Massage is always profoundly healing, and I included it as an integral part of my earlier Visionetics method. Now the addition of hypnosis has elevated the power of touch to new heights. External massage always reaches into internal areas, but this effect is vastly enhanced when direct suggestions are added. This is particularly true of the eyes because of their interconnection to the muscles of your shoulders, neck, and head. In fact, a full 20 percent of the functioning of your retinas originates in your shoulder muscles. As you massage these muscles you'll be energizing this layer of photo-sensitive cells so vital to the clarity of your vision at all distances.

Your minisessions will be the same as for the previous week. However, many people prefer to add some massage to the suggestions. I definitely encourage this. The more you massage, the more you open circulation into your eyes. This is a good thing you can't overdo!

By beginning your day with the overall shoulder-to-face massage, you'll be readying your entire body and mind, as well as your eyes, for the day ahead. You'll even find that the increased circulation into your face will make it look as well as feel younger. Hopefully you'll join the ranks of my clients who have forever made this massage a part of their daily lives.

There are seven parts to this first massage. The suggestions are essentially the same throughout, but it is important to tape them so that you don't have to think about them consciously. The more you lay your conscious mind to rest during the sessions, the deeper the suggestions will reach into your subconscious mind. So hypnotize yourself and then palm your eyes as you go on with the following:

o

"Feel your eyes letting go even more as you relax into the soothing darkness. . . . As they relax circulation into them increases. . . . Your eyes are alive with relaxation, circulation, and energy. . . . Your vision is regenerating. . . . In a few moments you will begin a massage that will dramatically increase circulation into your eyes and lenses and regenerate your vision even more. . . . Through this massage your near-point vision will become energized, relaxed, and clear. . . . Relax your hands down from your closed eyes now and sit so that you will be comfortable during the massage. Let your head relax forward and down. Bring your hands to your upper back and position them so that your fingers rest on either side on your spine, as far down your back as possible. . . . Begin stroking, hand over hand, out and over the top of your shoulders as you gradually massage your way up toward your neck. Pull those muscles out and up. Stroke all the way over your shoulder. One hand begins its stroke as the other is finished. Pull firmly, hand over hand. . . . With each stroke of your hands the muscles of your back are warming and relaxing, warming and relaxing. . . . Circulation is flowing into your spine and back muscles. More circulation flowing with each stroke of your hands. . . . Circulation and energy flowing up your spine, into your neck, and on into your visual system. . . . Your back and shoulders relax, and circulation and energy flow up into your visual system. It is rejuvenating as you massage. . . . Rejuvenating energy and circulation are flowing into the lenses of your eyes. . . . When you reach your neck, shorten your strokes and continue the massage, pulling the muscles away from your spine. Feel your neck muscles relaxing. . . . Warming and relaxing. . . . Circulation opening even more into your neck, your visual system, your eyes, the lenses of your eyes. Regenerating your lenses. . . . Your lenses are rich with circulation, energy, and nutrients. Your lenses are moist and flexible and adjust effortlessly to the shape necessary for clear vision at near-point. . . . Keep stroking and pulling those neck muscles away from your spine, gradually working your way up to the base of your skull. . . . If you find any lumpy or sensitive spots while working your way up your neck, give them some extra massaging attention. . . . Muscles relaxing, circulation flowing. . . . The effects of this massage go deep into your visual system. . . . Rejuvenating. . . . When you reach the base of your skull, reposition your hands so they are spread out over the back of your head and your thumbs are together at the center of the base of your skull, just above the top of your spine. Begin massaging in small, firm circular motions with your thumbs, and slowly work them apart, massaging all along that bony ridge out to the areas under your ears. . . . Let your breath seem to flow directly into the areas you are massaging. . . . You are massaging along a series of acupressure points, which release circulation and energy into your visual system, into your lenses themselves. . . . Circulation and energy flowing into your eyes, into your lenses. . . . Your lenses are energized and moist with circulation. Your lenses are youthful and flexible and easily adjust so you see clearly at nearpoint. . . . When you reach the areas under your ears, massage your way back to the center in those same small, firm circular motions. . . . Releasing even more healing energy and circulation into your visual system, into the lenses of your eyes. Add to the effect by letting your breath feel like it is flowing into the areas you are massaging. . . . Your lenses are rich with nutrients, circulation, and energy. They are rejuvenated and can easily adjust so you see clearly at nearpoint. . . . Moist and flexible. . . . After your thumbs come back together, begin massaging your scalp with your fingers. Press them firmly into your scalp and gently shake it loose from your skull. Work your way gradually over every part of your scalp, shaking and loosening. . . . Breathe deeply as you massage, and feel the circulation flooding into your scalp. It is also flowing into your eyes, into your lenses. . . . Your lenses are moist and flexible. . . . Massage in circles, up and down, back and forth. . . . It feels so good to open the circulation in your scalp. . . . Energy free now to flow into your visual system. . . . When you reach your forehead, spread your fingers over it. Shake it loose in the same way that you freed your scalp. . . . The relaxation, circulation, and energy in your forehead spreading into your eyes, into your lenses. . . . Moist, relaxed, regenerated. . . . Massage up and down and around in circles. . . . Now grasp your eyebrows at the inside corners with the thumb and index finger of each hand. Squeeze and massage your way back and forth across your eyebrows. . . . As you massage your eyebrows, they relax and circulation flows into them. . . . The circulation flows from your eyebrows into your eyes, into the lenses of your eyes. They are alive with relaxation and circulation and able to adjust so that you see clearly at nearpoint. . . . Your lenses are vibrantly healthy, moist, and flexible. . . . Now move on to the last step of this massage. Place your thumbs in the indentations in the bony ridges above your eyes just above their inside corners. Press in firm circular motions, and gradually work your way along the ridges to the outside corners of your eyes. Don't touch your eyes themselves, just massage along the ridges above them. You are massaging a series of acupressure points that release energy and circulation into your eyes. . . . When you reach the outside corners, change to your index fingers and massage your way along the bottom ridges to the inside corners of your eyes. . . . Energy and circulation are being released into your visual system, into your lenses. Your lenses are moist and flexible. . . . When you get to the inside corners, reverse your direction. Massage around and around. . . . Let your breath feel like it is flowing into the areas you are massaging. . . . Opening circulation and energy. . . . Your eyes and your mind are flexible and youthful. . . . It feels so good to be rejuvenating your vision. . . . Your nearpoint vision is absolutely capable of regenerating and clearing, and you know it. . . . The lenses of your eyes are alive with nutrients and circulation. Your lenses are youthful and flexible. They effortlessly adjust to a concave shape for near vision, and you see clearly up close. . . . You are completely confident of your rejuvenating vision. . . . Now finish massaging the bony ridge you are working on, and then palm your eyes. . . . Relax again into the soothing darkness. . . . Feel the warmth of your increased circulation, relaxation, and energy throughout your shoulders, neck, head, forehead, and eyes. . . . It feels so good. . . . You have dramatically increased the free flow of circulation and energy to all these areas. . . . Your muscles are relaxed and your circulation is rejuvenated and healthy. . . . Your lenses are moist and flexible. . . . Your lenses are effortlessly able to adjust for clear vision at close range. . . . You can see clearly at close range. . . . Feel the life and health in your eyes. . . . Know that your near vision is improving. . . . It feels so very good. . . . In a few moments I'll begin counting from one to five. At the subconscious level these numbers will allow your mind to accept and integrate even more deeply these positive changes that are occurring. At the conscious level these numbers will serve as signals that it is time to return to full waking alertness. By the number five you'll be fully alert, wonderfully refreshed, and seeing more clearly than before. One—a feeling of coming up. Let your breaths begin to deepen as you draw in energy. Two—still coming up. Feeling so completely relaxed and refreshed. Three—halfway up. Be aware of the feeling of circulation in your eyes. Your lenses are moist and flexible. You see clearly at close range. When you hear the next number, bring yourself all the way back to full conscious alertness. Four—all the way back. Feeling terrific. Keep your eyes closed as you take down your hands, and indulge in a yawn and a stretch. When you open your eyes blink softly and swing your head gently from side to side. Enjoy the energy, relaxation, and clarity of your vision."

o

Now you will understand why I was able to say that people invariably see better after this massage. It won't be long before your eyes and brain permanently retain the beneficial effects of this powerful relaxant and stimulant. If you keep all or part of it as a regular part of your life, you'll also find it wonderful for relieving general tension, headaches, and the blahs.

During the day try to get in three or more minisessions (see page 136) so that your subconscious will be reminded to keep the circulation flowing and your lenses flexible. You can simply palm during the minisessions, or you can choose some part of the massage session to do along with the suggestions. Then your later full session will be the Chinese acupressure massage. It is not quite as relaxing as the first one, but it is a powerful tonic and energizer for your entire visual system. It is an ancient technique that the Chinese government, in the last two decades, has instituted in regular daily use in schools, business, and industry.

Spend some time studying the illustrations on page 71 and locating all the acupressure points around your eyes before you perform the massage under hypnosis. You'll know you've found them when you experience what the Chinese call a "sour" feeling, which is something just short of pain. Some spots may be actually painful when you first find them, so be gentle but persistent in your massaging.

There are four parts to this massage; the first three are single spots and the fourth is the same series of points that you covered in the last step of the overall massage session. You'll use your thumbs on the first pair. They are just under your eyebrows on either side of the bridge of your nose. They are easy to find because there is a natural indentation there as well as sensitivity. You'll be massaging these points with firm circular motions. The second spots are just in from the corners of your eyes toward the bridge of your nose. You'll massage gently in and out on them with the thumb and forefinger of one hand. It is rare for anyone to experience tenderness on these points, but you'll most likely feel "gristly" little lumps. It is interesting to note that people who wear glasses often instinctively rub these areas after taking off their glasses. We have some good instincts!

The third points are sometimes difficult to find initially, but you'll know when you've found them because they tend to be quite sensitive. They are approximately one fingertip's width out from the bottom corners of your nose, along the edge of your cheekbone. Probe around with your index fingers until you find these sensitive indentations. You will be massaging these points with firm circular motions.

As you can see in the illustration, the fourth part of the massage covers a number of points above and below your eyes on the bony ridge surrounding them. Rather than working with each separately, you'll be stroking across the whole general area with the knuckle of your index finger. Curl your index finger and use the knuckle, not the smaller joint. Always stroke from the inside corners to the outside corners of the ridges. You want to use firm pressure, but not so much so that you stretch this delicate tissue.

After your induction, this massage will take approximately sixteen minutes. You'll rub each area for about one minute while absorbing the suggestions, going over the whole process four times. These acupressure points are so inherently powerful that a total of four minutes' attention to each is enough to activate them fully. While you can memorize the instructions, once again I recommend using a tape so your conscious mind can drift off out of the way.

After the acupressure massage there will be another short massage to bring all the energy and circulation you have released into your lenses even more. You will simply cup your hands together as if you were cupping them around a small bird. You'll gently press your hands more closed and then more round again. As you do this over and over, you'll imagine that it is your lenses that you are manipulating into alternating round and flat shapes. This is an amazing little massage in that you will quite literally feel the movement in your lenses. You would feel this even if you weren't hypnotized, but the effect will be even more profound because of your receptive state of mind.

Induce your hypnotic state and then absorb yourself in the following suggestion and directions:

o

"Palm your eyes for a moment. . . . Feel how quickly and deeply they let go into even deeper relaxation. . . . Wonderfully relaxed, circulation opening up already. . . . You know your lenses and your sight are rejuvenating. . . . You see more clearly at nearpoint with each passing day. . . . In a few moments you will begin a massage that will release even more energy and vitality into your visual system, into the lenses of your eyes. Not only will energy be released, but your subconscious will also fully accept and integrate within your visual system all the positive suggestions that will be

144 = HYPNOVISION

given. . . . Remove your hands from over your closed eyes now, and place your thumbs on the first acupressure points, the ones under your eyebrows just in from the bridge of your nose. Press firmly and rotate your thumbs in circles. As you massage, let it feel like your breath is flowing directly into these spots. . . . Healing energy and circulation are being released into your eyes. . . . With each rotation of your thumbs, more energy is released into your visual system, especially into the lenses of your eyes. . . . Your lenses are becoming rejuvenated. They are moist and flexible and can easily adjust so that you see clearly up close. . . . You can feel the healing energy being released. . . . Move on to the second points, pressing with the thumb and index finger of one hand just in from the corners of your eyes. Massage gently. . . . As you massage in and out on these points, healing energy is being released into your eyes. . . . Your ciliary muscles are relaxing as circulation flows into them. These muscles are fit and elastic and easily shift your lenses into the flatter, more concave shape for clear vision up close. . . . With each movement of your thumb and index finger, more rejuvenating energy is released into your ciliary muscles. . . . You can feel this massage stretching and toning your ciliary muscles. . . . Energized, toned, and relaxed. . . . Move on to the third points now, pressing on the sensitive indentations on the edges of your cheekbones a fingertip's width out from the bottom edge of your nose. Massage in small circular motions. . . . Healing energy is being released into your entire visual system. You can feel it, especially in the lenses of your eyes. Breathe right into the areas you are massaging. . . . The optic center of your brain clearly interprets nearpoint images. . . . You expect to see clearly at nearpoint, and you do. . . . Feel the healing energy pouring into your visual system. Into your lenses, into your ciliary muscles, into your retinas, down your optic nerves, and into the optic center of your brain. . . . It feels so good to rejuvenate your sight. . . . Move on now to stroking across the acupressure points on the ridges above and below your eyes. Use the knuckle of your index finger. Stroke from the inside corners out, top and bottom, top and bottom. . . . As your knuckles touch each of the acupressure points, healing energy is released. . . . Healthy, rejuvenating circulation flows into the lenses of your eyes. . . . Your lenses are moist and flexible. . . . Your lenses are rejuvenated. . . . You see clearly at close range. . . . It feels so good to know your sight is rejuvenating. . . . Relaxing, healing, energizing. . . ."

At this point, return to the beginning of the exercise and go through it three more times. Then continue.

"Now, as you feel the energy and circulation in your eyes and lenses, cup your hands together, fingertips of your right hand resting against the edge of your left thumb and fingertips of your left hand resting against the edge of your right little finger. Begin pressing your hands gently more flat and then rounding them out again. Your lenses feel and respond to this massage. You can feel them flattening and then rounding. . . . Flattening then rounding. . . . Breathe as you massage. Feel the massage in your lenses. . . . Your lenses are healthy, youthful, and flexible. . . . Your lenses are healthy, youthful, and flexible. . . . Your lenses easily shift their shape so you see clearly at all distances. . . . Your lenses are wonderfully flexible and change their shape when you shift focus, and you see clearly at all distances. . . . Your flexible lenses effortlessly adapt when you look up close, and you see clearly at nearpoint. . . . Your lenses are healthy, youthful, and flexible. . . . Let go of the massaging action and feel the circulation and life in your lenses. . . . Now palm your eyes and feel them relax even more into the soothing darkness. . . . The energy from the palms of your hands continues the release of energy into your visual system, into the lenses of your eyes. . . . Your lenses are healthy, moist, and flexible. . . . Your ciliary muscles are fit and elastic, and they easily shift your lenses into the shape necessary for clear vision at close range. . . . The optic center of your brain clearly interprets nearpoint images. . . . You can see clearly up close. . . . Your mind and your eyes are flexible and youthful. . . . Your vision is rejuvenated. . . . It feels so good to regain your clear near-point vision. . . . In a few moments I'll begin counting from one to five. At the subconscious level these numbers will allow your visual system and your lenses to integrate and benefit from the energy you have released into them even more fully. At the same time, these numbers will signal your conscious mind that it is time to return to full alertness. By the number five you'll be fully alert, refreshed, and seeing clearly at all distances. One—coming up. Your breaths deepening. Two—deeper breaths. Feeling energized and knowing your vision has improved even more. Three—halfway up. Notice how relaxed and moist with energy and circulation your eyes feel. Four—almost all the way back to full alertness. Feeling re-freshed and confident of your clear vision. When you hear the next number, bring yourself all the way back to full conscious alertness. Five—all the way back. Eyes alive with relaxation, circulation, and energy. Feeling wonderful. Take your hands down from your closed eyes and stretch and yawn. When you open your eyes blink softly as you swing your head gently from side to side. Enjoy the energy and clarity of your sight."

o

As with the first massage session, you'll most likely experience a burst of clarity in your nearpoint vision after you finish. By the end of this week of massage and suggestions, your lenses and visual system will be convinced that the rejuvenation process is taking place. With this firmly in your subconscious, you'll experience longer and more frequent periods of nearpoint clarity. Your eyes are getting the message!

I've seen a fair number of presbyopes reverse this condition in just two weeks. However, most people need more practice with seeing clearly before it becomes an ingrained pattern. That's what the next two weeks are about. The first one involves the constant shifting of your focus from far to near. The second moves on into putting everything together for actual reading. I'm sure you'll enjoy the process of your eyes continually gaining confidence in their rediscovered abilities.

WEEK THREE

Now we get down to the "work" sessions. Having said that, let me emphasize the importance of approaching them as play rather than work. Play is more natural and enjoyable than work, and we always learn new skills more quickly and competently if we develop them through play. Even though important work will be accomplished by your eyes, think of these exercises as vision games and have fun with them.

In the morning session you'll be gradually bringing your clear focus in nearer and nearer while your eyes also practice working as a coordinated team. In the later session your eyes will practice the skill of rapidly and completely shifting focus from the distance to the nearpoint. As you'll remember from Chapter 2, the teamwork required of your eyes to put together two slightly different images into one coherent one is known as fusion. The ability to shift focus from one distance to another is called accommodation. Once your eyes are reeducated in these two basic skills, they will be able to progress effortlessly to reading at nearpoint.

The morning exercise is called string fusion. It is a time-tested Bates technique that is dramatically enhanced by combining it with hypnosis. For it you will need a six-foot length of string, preferably the bright yellow kind sold at hardware stores. At one-foot intervals tie five knots in the string—it helps to fold the string in half and tie the middle knot first, so the rest are easier to space evenly. Unless you are working with a partner, you'll need to anchor one end to something just below your eye level. A doorknob or the back of a chair work well. You can either sit or stand as you do this exercise, just have the anchored end slightly lower than the one near you. Hold your end at the tip of your nose, and position yourself far enough back so that the string is taut.

As you can see in the illustration on page 101, the object is to see the optical illusion of two ghost strings crossing through the knot. You will be sliding your focused gaze up and down the string, seeing those ghost strings all along the way. Play with the string for a while in your conscious state of mind before you do it under hypnosis. This will give you an opportunity to gauge your present fusion skills as well as learn the exercise.

Begin your gaze focused on the string farthest away from you. This is the distance at which you already see clearly, so you'll see a strong image of the two strings coming together at the knot and stretching back toward you in the shape of an inverted V. Keep your eyes on the knot but be aware that on each of the ghost strings there are four knots coming in to you as well. Now slide your eyes in to the fourth knot. As you do you'll see the strings parting along with the point of your focus, and when you get to the knot you'll see two strings coming out of each end of it, as well as knots on them. Then, when you slide down to the middle knot, you'll see the illusion of a perfect X, two knots on each ghost string. Sliding in to the second knot, you'll find a reverse image of the fourth one. Then, bringing your focus all the way in to the first knot, you'll see a V extending out, four knots on each string.

Seeing this V coming out of the first knot is the primary goal. If you can already see it easily and clearly, your eyes are doing beautifully, and you can probably already read books without your glasses. But even if this is the case, don't skip this exercise. It will supply valuable practice and reinforcement of your regained visual skills. Most of you, on the other hand, will experience imperfect nearpoint fusion and clarity, especially at the first knot. By the end of the week, this will have cleared up and your eyes will be functioning well at nearpoint. Without the use of hypnosis it can take months of work to develop nearpoint fusion skills, but the power of hypnosis has transformed this into a quick and easy adjustment on the part of your eyes.

So, ready to *play* now, have your fusion string set up, hypnotize yourself, and go on with the following:

o

"Palm your eyes. Feel them immediately relax into the soothing darkness. . . . Your eyes are relaxed and healthy. . . . Your vision is rapidly rejuvenating. There is an open flow of circulation into the lenses of your eyes. Your lenses are moist and flexible. Your ciliary muscles are fit and elastic. Your ciliary muscles effortlessly shift your youthful, flexible lenses into the flatter, more concave shape for nearpoint vision, and you see clearly. You see clearly at all distances. . . . Activate your imagination now, and imagine that you are looking down the fusion string, focused on the knot farthest away from you. You can see it clearly as well as the two ghost strings coming in to you in the shape of an inverted V. On each ghost string are four evenly spaced knots. Now imagine sliding your gaze in along the string to the fourth knot. The strings part as you move your focus down them. You see the knot clearly, one knot on each of the strings in the distance and three knots on the ones coming in to you. Visualize sliding your gaze in to the middle knot and seeing a perfect X, two knots on each of the ghost strings. As you visualize this exercise, your ciliary muscles and lenses actually go through the motions that create clear sight. The muscles perfectly shift your flexible lenses into a flatter, more concave shape as you slide your imagined gaze in to the second knot, seeing the strings part and observing the three knots on the distant strings and the single knot on the strings coming in to you. Your lenses and muscles again perform perfectly as you imagine sliding your gaze in to the first knot. You see it perfectly clearly, as well as observing the four knots on the ghost strings in the form of a V. Good. Let the image fade and relax into the darkness again. . . . Your lenses are youthful, moist, and flexible, and they adapt perfectly to the flatter, more concave shape necessary for clear vision up close. In a few moments you will open your eyes and begin using the fusion string. When you do, your flexible lenses and fit ciliary muscles will perform flawlessly, and you will see clearly at all distances. You will remain hypnotized when you open your eyes, but you will be alert, balanced, and steady. . . . Take your palms down from your eyes, and give your eyes a few moments to begin readjusting to the light while they are behind your closed lids.

Feeling confident of the flexibility of your lenses. . . . Open your eyes now, blinking softly and gently swinging your head from side to side. . . . Position yourself with one end of the fusion string at the tip of your nose. The string is taut between you and its anchor. Look down the string and focus your gaze on the last string. Breathe and blink as you see it clearly, aware of the two ghost strings coming in toward you, each with four knots on it. Take in a breath and let it out as you slide your eyes down to the fourth knot, blinking as you observe the strings opening as you slide your gaze down. You see the fourth knot clearly and are aware of the two strings coming out the top of it, each with one knot, and the two longer strings coming in to you, each with three knots. . . . The closer you bring in your focus, the more your lenses adapt to a flatter, more concave shape and you see clearly. . . . Another nice breath in, exhaling and blinking as you slide in to the middle knot. Keep blinking and breathing as you see a perfect X at the knot and observe the four strings coming out of it, each with two knots. The farther in you slide your eyes, the more your lenses change into a flatter, more concave shape and you see clearly. Take in a deeper breath and let it out, blinking, as you slide in to the second knot, enjoying the image of the strings parting and seeing the second knot clearly, aware of the knots on the ghost strings. Your lenses are moist and flexible, and you see clearly at all distances. Take in a still-deeper breath, and exhale and blink as you easily slide your focus in along the string to the first knot. Breathe and blink as you see it clearly. The two ghost strings extend into the distance in a perfect V shape, and you are aware that each has four knots. . . . Now take in another of those deep breaths, and let it out, blinking, while you slide your focus smoothly and continuously out on the string all the way to the last knot. See the string part in front of you and cross at each knot while you slide all the way to the last one. . . . Now come back just as you did before. A breath in, let it out, and slide in to the fourth knot. Eyes moving effortlessly, blinking frequently. See the knots on the ghost strings. Another inhalation and another exhalation as you slide in to the third knot. Strings parting, seeing a perfect X at the knot, ghost strings coming in and out each with two knots. You see so effortlessly and so clearly. The closer in you bring your focus, the more your lenses shift into a flatter, more concave shape and you see clearly. Another breath, blink and exhale as you slide in to the second knot. You see it clearly. It's enjoyable to bring your focus in closer. A deeper breath in. Blink as you exhale and slide in to the first knot. Lenses flexible. You see the first knot clearly, and you are aware of the ghost strings extending out in the shape of a V, each with four knots. Neck, shoulders, face, and eyes relaxed as you clearly see the first knot. Flexible lenses adapting to the flatter, more concave shape necessary for clear nearpoint vision. . . . Once more take in a deep breath and let it out as you slide all the way back down the string to the last knot. Blink and enjoy how you move the strings and see the knots and crossing strings clearly as you slide out. See the last knot clearly. In a few moments you will be sliding your gaze back down to the first knot. As you do, your fit ciliary muscles will effortlessly shift your flexible lenses into a flatter, almost concave, shape so that you will see clearly as you move your gaze in. Take in a deep breath and let it out as you slide all the way in to the first knot. Blinking. Flexible lenses shifting shape. Seeing clearly. Shoulders, neck, face, and eyes relaxed. See the first knot clearly, two strings with four knots extending into the distance in a perfect V. . . . Another deep breath and another smooth slide all the way back to the last knot. Blink and enjoy how well you do this. See the last knot clearly, two strings coming in to you each with four knots. . . . Now come back in one knot at a time again. An inhalation and then an exhalation as you slide back to the fourth knot. Blinking, relaxing. Seeing clearly. The more you bring your focus in close, the more your lenses change into a flatter, more concave shape. Breathe in and let the breath out as you easily slide in to the middle knot. Strings parting as you slide. The X and the knots are clear. The closer you focus the more your lenses shift into a concave shape and you see clearly. Shoulders, neck, face, and eyes relaxed. Breathe in and then exhale as you effortlessly slide in to the second knot. Seeing it clearly, aware of all the knots. When you slide in to the first knot, your lenses will shift into an even flatter, almost concave, shape and you will see the knot clearly. Inhale and blink as you exhale and slide in to the first knot. So effortlessly, so clearly. Good. . . . Now put down the string, close your eyes, and palm them once again. . . . Feel your eyes instantly relaxing into the soothing darkness. . . . In a moment I'll count from three down to one. With each number down, experience that downward sensation that brings you into even deeper hypnotic relaxation. Three, every muscle, nerve, and cell relaxing down. Two, deeper down, more pleasantly relaxed. When you hear the next number, double your relaxation with a wave of letting go or a deep sinking sensation. One, doubling your relaxation. Deeply, wonderfully relaxed. . . . Your eyes are relaxed and circulation flows freely into them. . . . Rejuvenating circulation, energy, and relaxation are flowing into the lenses of your eyes. . . . The exercise you have just completed has taught your ciliary muscles and lenses to adapt to nearpoint so that you see clearly. Each time you practice the exercise your nearpoint vision improves. . . . Your mind and your eyes are youthful and flexible, and you see clearly up close. . . . It is enjoyable to rejuvenate your near vision. . . . Your lenses are moist and flexible, and they adapt easily into the flatter, more concave shape necessary for clear vision. You see clearly up close. . . . You expect to see clearly up close and you do. . . . You are young in spirit, and this is reflected by the flexibility of your vision. It feels so good to rejuvenate your vision. You see clearly at nearpoint. It feels so good. You are completely confident of your ability to see clearly up close. . . . In a few moments I'll count from one to five. With each number up your subconscious will more fully accept and integrate every positive suggestion that has been made. At the conscious level these numbers will serve as reminders that it is time to return to full alertness. By the number five you'll be fully alert, wonderfully refreshed, and confident of the clarity of your near vision. One—coming up. Let your breaths deepen. Energy starting to increase. Two—coming up more. So relaxed, energized, and confident. Three—halfway up. Be aware of the pleasant feeling of moisture and circulation in your eyes. So refreshed and healthy. Four—almost all the way back. Confident that your near vision is rejuvenating. When you hear the next number, bring yourself all the way back to full conscious alertness. Five—all the way back. Feeling terrific. Take your hands down from your closed eyes. Enjoy a stretch and a yawn. When you open your eyes, blink softly and swing your head gently from side to side. Enjoy the vitality and clarity of your vision."

o

You will see the beneficial effects of this exercise all during your day. Your eye muscles are fit and coordinated and your lenses well practiced at shifting focus. You'll find that with each passing day you can see more clearly up close for longer periods of time. Don't forget to take time out three times during your day for the minisessions on page 136. These will further reinforce the ability of your lenses to integrate the work you have done as well as provide them with extra doses of rejuvenating circulation.

The morning session asked your eyes to make gradual adjustments in focusing. The later one builds on that ability and extends your skills to making large and rapid shifts of accommodation. You'll be moving your focus from the distance to the nearpoint with the same clarity at each that you experienced before you needed reading glasses. This is yet another exercise that is slow and laborious in the optometric and Bates approaches but quick and easy with HypnoVision.

Now remove or make a copy of the two charts provided in the back of the book. As you can see, they are identical except for size. Place the large one at eye level (decide if you will sit or stand for this exercise) on a well-illuminated wall. You'll be sitting or standing about ten or fifteen feet back from it, a distance at which you can see it clearly. You'll be holding the small card in front of you at reading distance. While hypnotized, you will be shifting your vision from the clear distant letters in to the smaller versions of them. If you can already read the small letters you'll be reinforcing this skill, and if not you'll be developing it. As you progress through the letters, your nearpoint vision will become increasingly clear.

Make yourself comfortable sitting or lying down, hypnotize yourself, and continue with the following script:

o

"Palm your eyes and relax into the soothing darkness. . . . Your lenses are moist and flexible. . . . Rejuvenating circulation flows freely into the lenses of your eyes. . . . Your lenses are nourished, moist, and flexible. . . . You are youthful and flexible in your mind and in your vision. . . . Your ciliary muscles are fit and elastic. . . . Your lenses adjust effortlessly into the flatter, more concave shape for near vision, and you see clearly. . . . Every time you practice shifting your focus from far to near, your lenses learn more fully to see clearly up close. . . . You enjoy the process of rejuvenating your near vision. . . . Use your imagination now and visualize doing the accommodation exercise. Imagine seeing a white piece of paper in the distance. On it the letter *F* is very black and very clear. Notice how the black contrasts with the white. In a moment you will imagine looking in at a small *F* on a white card in your hand. When you do, your ciliary muscles and lenses will adjust just as if you were really seeing the letter. Study just how the big *F* looks. And now imagine shifting your focus in to the small *F* on a card in your hand. You see it just as clearly as you did the large *F*. Imagine looking into this distance again and this time seeing a black *O* on a white piece of paper. Observe the contrast between the black and the white. Imagine shifting your vision to the white card in your hand and seeing a small *O*, very black and clear against the white background. When you imagined shifting in to the near *O*, your ciliary muscles and lenses adjusted into the proper shape for clear near vision. Visualize looking back out at the white paper and this time seeing a black *E* on it.

Observe the four lines that make it up. Imagine looking at the card in front of you and clearly seeing a small black *E*. Your ciliary muscles and lenses adjusted, and your brain interpreted the *E* clearly. In your mind's eye look into the distance once more and see a large black *M*. See the black in contrast to the white. Imagine looking to the card in your hand and clearly seeing a small black *M* against the white background. Your lenses and ciliary muscles actually shifted and the optic center of your brain clearly interpreted the *M*. . . . Let the images fade away and relax into the soothing darkness once again. In a few moments you'll begin this exercise with your physical eyes, and they will adjust just as well as when you imagined seeing clearly. You will remain hypnotized when you open your eyes, but you will be alert, steady, and balanced. Your lenses are rejuvenated, moist, and flexible, and you see clearly at nearpoint. . . . Remaining pleasantly hypnotized, relax your hands down from your closed eyes. Give them a few moments to begin readjusting to the light behind your closed lids. Then, when you open your eyes, blink them softly as you gently swing your head from side to side. . . . Take up a position where you are eye level with the large chart, standing back at a comfortable distance and seeing it clearly, and hold the small chart in front of you at reading distance. Look at the first letter in the first row on the far chart, the *F*. As you observe the black *F* against the white background, be aware of the three black lines that make it up. Close your eyes and vividly remember the *F*. You will see the small *F* just as clearly as the larger one. Your ciliary muscles will adjust your lenses so that you will see it clearly. Take in a breath and, as you let it out, shift your focus to the small *F* on the near chart. Blink softly as you observe it. Be aware of the blackness of the three lines that make it up against the white background. . . . Look back to the far chart to the second letter, the *O*. Observe its shape, it is taller than it is wide, and the contrast between the black and the white. Close your eyes and remember the *O*. Imagine it clearly. Black against white, the white in the center. Take in a breath and exhale and blink as you look in to the small *O*. Fit ciliary muscles adjusting your flexible lenses. You can see the black in contrast to the white and the white center of the *O*. Look back out now to the *E*. Study its four black lines in contrast to the white background. Close your eyes and remember the *E*. When you look at the small *E*, you will see it just as clearly. Breathe in, exhale, blink, and look in to the small *E*. Its four black lines stand out against the white background. Shoulders, neck, face, and eyes relaxed. Look out to the last letter of the first row, the *M*. Note how the four black lines that make it up are in different positions than for the *E*. Close your eyes and remember the *M* vividly. Your lenses are moist and flexible and will shift into the shape necessary to see the small *M*. Inhale, exhale, and look in at the small *M*. Your lenses adjusting better every time you look in. See the black *M* against the white background, noticing each of its four lines. . . . Look back out to the first line of the second row, the *B*. See the straight line and the two curved lines that make it up. Black on white. Close your eyes and remember the black *B* against a white background. Vividly see the white centers of each half of the *B*. Your lenses are youthful and flexible, and you will be able to see this *B* just as clearly at nearpoint. Inhale, exhale, and blink as you shift in to the small *B*. Very black against the white background, the white centers of each half standing out clearly. You see the *B* clearly. Look back out to the *J*. Study it, see the contrast. Close your eyes and remember the *J* clearly. Inhale and then exhale as you open your eyes to look at the small *J* in front of you. Lenses adjusting so that you see it clearly. Black on white. Look back out to the *K*. Observe its lines and the contrast of black against white. Close your eyes and visualize the *K* just as clearly. Every time you adjust your focus to close range, your lenses shift more fully than before. A breath in and then let it out as you look to the small *K*. Blinking and seeing the black lines against the white background. Your near vision is improving. Look back out to the last letter of the second row, the *P*. See it very clearly against the white background. Your eyes are relaxed and energetic, they enjoy this exercise. Close your eyes and remember the *P*. Your lenses are flexible and enjoy adjusting for clear vision at close range. Then breathe in another breath and then exhale as you look in to the near *P*. You see it so clearly, black against white. Each shift more clear than the one before it. Look back out to the first letter of the third row, the *A*. Be aware of the three lines that make it up. You know you will see it just as clearly up close. Close your eyes and visualize the *A*, very black against a white background, the white center standing out. Your lenses are rejuvenated and flexible and can adjust so you see this *A* clearly at close range. Inhale, then exhale as you shift in to the near *A*. Blinking. The optic center of your brain clearly interprets the *A*. Its white center stands out against its black lines. Look back to the far chart, to the *C*. Study its curve. You are confident of seeing it just as clearly in your mind's eye and at close range. Close your eyes and clearly visualize the *C*. So black against the white background. What you can visualize you can see clearly. Breathe in, then blink as you exhale and focus on the near *C*. It is so clear. With each practice at accommodation your lenses function better and you see more clearly. Look out to the distant *D*, noting its straight line and its curve. Very black against the white background. Close your eyes and remember the black *D* against the white background. The optic center of your brain remembers the *D* and will see it just as clearly when you look at the small *D*. Breathe in, exhale, and blink as you focus clearly on the near *D*. It is very black against the white background. Shoulders, neck, face, and eyes relaxed. Look up and out now to the last letter of the third row, the *X*. Study these black crossed lines. The optic center of your brain is memorizing the *X*. Close your eyes and visualize the *X*. So black against a white background. The optic center of your brain remembers the *X* clearly and will interpret the small *X* as clearly. A breath in and an exhalation as you look in to the small *X*. Blink. You see the two crossing black lines so clearly. The optic center of your brain interprets the *X* clearly. Look back out to the first letter of the last row, the Q. Study its shape and the contrast of black against white. Close your eyes and remember the Q. Your lenses are moist and elastic and will adjust so that you see the Q just as clearly at close range. Inhale, and exhale and blink as you look in to the small Q. Ciliary muscles adjusting your lenses and you see the black Q clearly against the white background. Your vision is energetic yet relaxed. Look back out at the R, noting its straight and curved lines. Memorize the R. Close your eyes and clearly visualize the R, so black against the white background. You see it clearly in your mind, and when you look at the small R your lenses will adjust so that you will see it clearly. Breathe in, let it out as you look at the near R. Blinking. The black R is so vivid against the white background. You see its straight and curved lines. The R is clear. Look back out now to the G. See the contrast and memorize the G. The optic center of your brain is memorizing the G. Close your eyes and remember the G. The optic center of your brain will interpret the near G this clearly. Breathe in, and exhale and blink as you focus on the small G. Your lenses adjust to bring it in clearly, and the optic center of your brain interprets the G as clearly. Your lenses are energized and flexible. You see the G clearly. Look back out now to the last letter, the S. Notice its black curves against the white background. Close your eyes and visualize the S. Very black against a contrasting white background. The optic center of your brain remembers it clearly and will see the near S just as clearly. When you shift your vision in to the near S, your ciliary muscles will adjust your lenses into a flatter, more concave shape and you will see the S clearly. A deep breath in, and let it out as you focus clearly on the near S. Ciliary muscles adjusting your lenses. Blinking. Optic center of your brain clearly interpreting the S. Good. . . . Now go through the whole process once more, much more quickly this time and without the pause to visualize the letters. Start with the first letter on the far chart, the F. See it clearly, then shift your vision in to the near F, seeing it just as clearly. Keep on going, letter by letter, in and out. . . . Your lenses are moist, healthy, and flexible. They adjust shape as you focus on the near letters, and you see them clearly. . . . Breathing and blinking. . . . The optic center of your brain memorizes each letter in the distance and then interprets the small letters just as clearly. . . . It's fun and effortless to shift in and out. . . . Your lenses are moist, healthy, and flexible. . . . Your lenses adjust so you see clearly at close range. . . . Your lenses are healthy and flexible and you see clearly up close. . . . Effortlessly shifting in and out. . . . Seeing clearly at all distances. . . . You see just as clearly at nearpoint as you do in the distance. . . . Effortlessly shifting in and out. . . . Your sight is rejuvenated and clear at all distances. . . . Finish up with the whole chart. . . . Make yourself comfortable sitting or lying down and palm your eyes now. Feel them relax instantly into the soothing darkness. . . . They've had a wonderful workout. They feel fit and healthy. . . . In a few moments I'll count down from three to one. Experience a downward sensation with each number and feel yourself entering even more deeply into the hypnotic state. Three—relaxing as you move down. Two—deeper down, deeper relaxed. When you hear the next number, double your relaxation. One—doubling your relaxation. . . . So deeply and wonderfully relaxed. . . . Each time you do this exercise you see more clearly at nearpoint. . . . Your vision is relaxed and clear. . . . There is a free and open flow of circulation into the lenses of your eyes. . . . Your lenses are healthy and rejuvenated. . . . Your mind and your lenses are youthful and flexible. . . . Every time you practice focusing up close you see more clearly. . . . It feels so good to regain your clear nearpoint vision. . . . You are completely confident of your clear nearpoint vision. . . . Your eyes are relaxed and refreshed. . . . Your eyes are relaxed and refreshed, and you see clearly up close. . . . Your lenses are rejuvenated and you see clearly up close. . . . Your eyes are relaxed and refreshed. . . . In a few moments I'll begin counting from one to five. With each number up your visual system will more fully accept and integrate all the benefits of the exercise you have just done. At the same time these numbers will signal your conscious mind that it is time to return to full alertness. By the number five you'll be fully alert, wonderfully relaxed and refreshed, seeing clearly at all distances. One—a feeling of coming up, your breathing deepening and your energy flowing. Two—coming up. Feeling so relaxed and refreshed. Confident of your clear nearpoint vision. Three—halfway up. You can feel the energy and circulation in your lenses. You know you see clearly up close. Four— almost all the way back. It feels so good to be regenerating your vision. When you hear the next number, bring yourself all the way back to full conscious alertness. Five—all the way back. Feeling so good, so regenerated. Uncover your closed eyes and let them begin readjusting to the light behind your lids. Take in a deep breath and stretch and yawn. When you open your eyes, blink them softly and gently swing your head from side to side. Know that you've regenerated your near vision, and enjoy it."

o

Each day you do the fusion and accommodation exercises, your lenses will regain both the confidence and the ability to again see clearly at nearpoint. You'll find yourself resorting to reading glasses less and less. Your lenses are becoming athletic and vital again and shedding the need for crutches. You'll see this revitalization process spilling over into other areas of your life. You're regaining your youth, enjoy it!

All that's left to do now is to teach your eyes some simple reading skills. When your lenses began to lose their flexibility, you unconsciously created tension throughout your visual system. Clear vision occurs when your eyes are in a state of dynamic relaxation. Effort and tension freeze up the visual process both physiologically and mentally. During the next week you'll learn to read in a way that restores the spontaneous coordination between your eyes and mind while your lenses continue to develop more flexibility.

WEEK FOUR

The single biggest obstacle I encountered when teaching my clients to read at nearpoint with the Bates techniques was their belief system. Even when they were successfully reading fine print, I'd hear exclamations of "I can't believe I'm actually reading this!" And then, *poof*, the clarity would vanish. They had the flexibility back in their lenses, a good flow of circulation, and all the necessary skills, but they still often never fully regained their reading ability because they plain and simple didn't believe they were capable of it.

You won't have this problem because you've been restructuring your belief system at the subconscious level for three weeks now. You've also spent this same amount of time reestablishing circulation and flexibility in your lenses. Quite some time ago I read that scientists have determined that it takes three weeks for habit changes to be fully integrated within a person's psyche. I concur, especially when the hypnotic process is used and the changes are accepted at the subconscious level. Your eyes and your mind are now completely primed for clear and effortless nearpoint vision.

Your full sessions this week will be spent doing exactly what you picked up this book to accomplish, reading at nearpoint. The only difference, of course, is that this week you'll be reading while hypnotized. The reading material consists of skills and suggestions for nearpoint clarity. As you practice reading, your visual system will relax and let go of the last vestiges of tension and negative expectancy that have hampered your vision since the time you first began to experience difficulty at nearpoint.

The morning session will allow your eyes to gradually loosen up and focus on decreasing sizes of print. Then, in the later session, when your eyes are warmed up by a full day of use, you will progress more rapidly through the ever smaller lines of print. Your lenses will continue to develop their flexibility while your mind learns how to attain the relaxation necessary for clear vision. In between the full sessions you'll do the same minisessions that you've been working with all along.

Because you'll be reading the suggestions and instructions, you won't need to tape them. However, some people have found that they respond so well to spoken suggestions that they prefer them for these sessions as well. Also, if you feel that going on to actual reading will be a big step for you, you may want to tape the sessions for the reinforcement of the written suggestions. Whichever method you chose, you will be reading for about fifteen minutes. And, of course, you will be reading without your glasses!

Memorize the first section of the session as you will be doing it while palming. When you are finished with it, open your eyes and begin reading.

Here we go. Induce your hypnotic state and then think the following:

o

"As I palm my eyes they relax deeply. . . . My lenses are youthful and flexible. . . . Circulation flows into the lenses of my eyes and keeps them nourished and flexible. . . . My lenses adjust into a flatter, more concave shape for near vision, and I see clearly. . . . When I read at nearpoint I concentrate on the whiteness in and around the letters. . . . As I remain aware of the whiteness, the black print stands out clearly. . . . I see clearly up close. . . . When I open my eyes they will function optimally and I will see clearly up close. . . . Even with my eyes open I will remain in a pleasant, deep state of hypnosis. . . ."

o

Open your eyes now, blinking and swinging your head from side to side. Begin reading now, and your vision will remain clear as the print becomes smaller:

As I read I let my eyes slide under the words. I am very aware of the white spaces in and around the lines of print. I allow the whiteness to seem so bright that it appears to glow. I breathe evenly, blink regularly, and slide my vision under the lines of print. The black letters appear very dark in contrast to the whiteness. The whiteness in and around the black letters seems to glow brightly. My lenses are moist and flexible. They effortlessly adjust so that I see clearly up close. I am far more interested in the whiteness than in the black letters. The black letters appear very clearly in contrast to the whiteness. I see the black letters clearly as I effortlessly slide my gaze under them. My lenses are flexible and moist. As I read my entire visual system remains relaxed. It is easy and effortless to see clearly up close. I breathe and blink as I read, and my vision remains relaxed. The smaller the print becomes, the more my lenses adjust so that I see clearly up close. I see clearly up close. My nearpoint vision is regenerated.

As I read I let my eyes slide under the words. I am very aware of the white spaces in and around the lines of print. I allow the whiteness to seem so bright that it appears to glow. I breathe evenly, blink regularly, and slide my vision under the lines of print. The black letters appear very dark in contrast to the whiteness. The whiteness in and around the black letters seems to glow brightly. My lenses are moist and flexible. They effortlessly adjust so that I see clearly up close. I am far more interested in the whiteness than in the black letters. The black letters appear very clearly in contrast to the whiteness. I see the black letters clearly as I effortlessly slide my gaze under them. My lenses are flexible and moist. As I read my entire visual system remains relaxed. It is easy and effortless to see clearly up close. I breathe and blink as I read, and my vision remains relaxed. The smaller the print becomes, the more my lenses adjust so that I see clearly up close. I see clearly up close. My nearpoint vision is regenerated.

As I read I let my eyes slide under the words. I am very aware of the white spaces in and around the lines of print. I allow the whiteness to seem so bright that it appears to glow. I breathe evenly, blink regularly, and slide my vision under the lines of print. The black letters appear very dark in contrast to the whiteness. The whiteness in and around the black letters seems to glow brightly. My lenses are moist and flexible. They effortlessly adjust so that I see clearly up close. I am far more interested in the whiteness than in the black letters. The black letters appear very clearly in contrast to the whiteness. I see the black letters clearly as I effortlessly slide my gaze under them. My lenses are flexible and moist. As I read my entire visual system remains relaxed. It is easy and effortless to see clearly up close. I breathe and blink as I read, and my vision remains relaxed. The smaller the print becomes, the more my lenses adjust so that I see clearly up close. I see clearly up close. My nearpoint vision is regenerated.

As I read I let my eyes slide under the words. I am very aware of the white spaces in and around the lines of print. I allow the whiteness to seem so bright that it appears to glow. I breathe evenly, blink regularly, and slide my vision under the lines of print. The black letters appear very dark in contrast to the whiteness. The whiteness in and around the black letters seems to glow brightly. My lenses are moist and flexible. They effortlessly adjust so that I see clearly up close. I am far more interested in the whiteness than in the black letters. The black letters appear very clearly in contrast to the whiteness. I see the black letters clearly as I effortlessly slide my gaze under them. My lenses are flexible and moist. As I read my entire visual system remains relaxed. It is easy and effortless to see clearly up close. I breathe and blink as I read, and my vision remains relaxed. The smaller the print becomes, the more my lenses adjust so that I see clearly up close. I see clearly up close. My nearpoint vision is regenerated.

As I read I let my eyes slide under the words. I am very aware of the white spaces in and around the lines of print. I allow the whiteness to seem so bright that it appears to glow. I breathe evenly, blink regularly, and slide my vision under the lines of print. The black letters appear very dark in contrast to the whiteness. The whiteness in and around the black letters seems to glow brightly. My lenses are moist and flexible. They effortlessly adjust so that I see clearly up close. I am far more interested in the whiteness than in the black letters. The black letters appear very clearly in contrast to the whiteness. I see the black letters clearly as I effortlessly slide my gaze under them. My lenses are flexible and moist. As I read my entire visual system remains relaxed. It is easy and effortless to see clearly up close. I breathe and blink as I read, and my vision remains relaxed. The smaller the print becomes, the more my lenses adjust so that I see clearly up close. I see clearly up close. My nearpoint vision is regenerated.

As I read I let my eyes slide under the words. I am very aware of the white spaces in and around the lines of print. I allow the whiteness to seem so bright that it appears to glow. I breathe evenly, blink regularly, and slide my vision under the lines of print. The black letters appear very dark in contrast to the whiteness. The whiteness in and around the black letters seems to glow brightly. My lenses are moist and flexible. They effortlessly adjust so that I see clearly up close. I am far more interested in the whiteness than in the black letters. The black letters appear very clearly in contrast to the whiteness. I see the black letters clearly as I effortlessly slide my gaze under them. My lenses are flexible and moist. As I read my entire visual system remains relaxed. It is easy and effortless to see clearly up close. I breathe and blink as I read, and my vision remains relaxed. The smaller the print becomes, the more my lenses adjust so that I see clearly up close. I see clearly up close. My nearpoint vision is regenerated.

As I read I let my eyes slide under the words. I am very aware of the white spaces in and around the lines of print. I allow the whiteness to seem so bright that it appears to glow. I breathe evenly, blink regularly, and slide my vision under the lines of print. The black letters appear very dark in contrast to the whiteness. The whiteness in and around the black letters seems to glow brightly. My lenses are moist and flexible. They effortlessly adjust so that I see clearly up close. I am far more interested in the whiteness than in the black letters. The black letters appear very clearly in contrast to the whiteness. I see the black letters clearly as I effortlessly slide my gaze under them. My lenses are flexible and moist. As I read my entire visual system remains relaxed. It is easy and effortless to see clearly up close. I breathe and blink as I read, and my vision remains relaxed. The smaller the print becomes, the more my lenses adjust so that I see clearly up close. I see clearly up close. My nearpoint vision is regenerated.

As I read I let my eyes slide under the words. I am very aware of the white spaces in and around the lines of print. I allow the whiteness to seem so bright that it appears to glow. I breathe evenly, blink regularly, and slide my vision under the lines of print. The black letters appear very dark in contrast to the whiteness. The whiteness in and around the black letters seems to glow brightly. My lenses are moist and flexible. They effortlessly adjust so that I see clearly up close. I am far more interested in the whiteness than in the black letters. The black letters appear very clearly in contrast to the whiteness. I see the black letters clearly as I effortlessly slide my gaze under them. My lenses are flexible and moist. As I read my entire visual system remains relaxed. It is easy and effortless to see clearly up close. I breathe and blink as I read, and my vision remains relaxed. The smaller the print becomes, the more my lenses adjust so that I see clearly up close. I see clearly up close. My nearpoint vision is regenerated.

After reading all the material over and over for about fifteen minutes, during which time your vision will become clearer and clearer,

close your eyes and palm them. Think the following suggestions to
yourself:

o

"Every day in every way my sight is becoming more healthy
and vigorous. . . . Every time I practice reading I see the print
more clearly. . . . My visual system is relaxed. . . . Circulation
and nutrients flow freely into my lenses. . . . My lenses are
rejuvenated and healthy, and I see clearly up close. . . . My
eyes are relaxed and youthful. . . . My eyes are relaxed and
rejuvenated, and I see clearly at nearpoint."

o

Remain palming as long as you like, then count yourself up into full
alertness, feeling rested, refreshed, and confident of your ability to
see clearly at nearpoint.

Even if the smallest print is not clear to you in the beginning of each
hypnosis session, just keep sliding your eyes under it and focusing
your awareness on the whiteness. This attitude of relaxation and
lack of effort will quickly pay off. Once you overcome the bad habit
of straining to see, your whole visual system will perform with the
relaxed spontaneity that produces the clearest vision. This will also,
of course, enhance the ability of your lenses to adjust to the proper
shape for clear reading. Before long you'll be reading even the
smallest paragraph of print with ease and clarity.

During the day you'll be reinforcing the whole process with the
minisessions on page 136. If you haven't been including a little
massage along with them, this would be a good time to reinstate this
habit. The more relaxation and circulation you create, the easier
your eyes will adapt to effortless reading.

Your reading for the later session is similar to the first except that
the print will become smaller with each sentence rather than each
paragraph. There are only eight sentences, so you'll be reading
them over and over for the fifteen minutes. These repetitions will
give your lenses plenty of opportunity for adjustment and will send
the suggestions even deeper into your subconscious.

Once again hypnotize yourself, palm your eyes, and think the following suggestions to yourself before proceeding with the reading:

o

"My eyes are wonderfully relaxed. . . . My lenses are flexible. . . . My ciliary muscles shift my lenses into a flatter, more concave shape when I focus up close, and I see clearly. . . . Reading up close is easy and effortless. . . . My lenses are moist and flexible. . . . They effortlessly adjust shape so that I see clearly up close. . . . My entire visual system remains relaxed as I read. . . . I concentrate on the whiteness as I read, and the print is very black in contrast. . . . My lenses are vibrant with healthy circulation. . . . My lenses are moist and flexible and effortlessly adjust so that I see clearly up close. . . . I will remain in a pleasant, deep state of hypnosis when I open my eyes and read."

o

Open your eyes now and read the following eight sentences over and over for fifteen minutes:

As I read I slide my eyes under the lines of print and concentrate on the whiteness.

As I read I slide my eyes under the lines of print and concentrate on the whiteness.

As I read I slide my eyes under the lines of print and concentrate on the whiteness.

As I read I slide my eyes under the lines of print and concentrate on the whiteness.

As I read I slide my eyes under the lines of print and concentrate on the whiteness.

As I read I slide my eyes under the lines of print and concentrate on the whiteness.

As I read I slide my eyes under the lines of print and concentrate on the whiteness.

As I read I slide my eyes under the lines of print and concentrate on the whiteness.

The white under, around, and in the black print is so white that it seems to glow brightly.

The white under, around, and in the black print is so white that it seems to glow brightly.

The white under, around, and in the black print is so white that it seems to glow brightly.

The white under, around, and in the black print is so white that it seems to glow brightly.

The white under, around, and in the black print is so white that it seems to glow brightly.

The white under, around, and in the black print is so white that it seems to glow brightly.

The white under, around, and in the black print is so white that it seems to glow brightly.

The white under, around, and in the black print is so white that it seems to glow brightly.

As I read I breathe evenly, blink regularly, and my entire visual system remains relaxed.

As I read I breathe evenly, blink regularly, and my entire visual system remains relaxed.

As I read I breathe evenly, blink regularly, and my entire visual system remains relaxed.

As I read I breathe evenly, blink regularly, and my entire visual system remains relaxed.

As I read I breathe evenly, blink regularly, and my entire visual system remains relaxed.

As I read I breathe evenly, blink regularly, and my entire visual system remains relaxed.

As I read I breathe evenly, blink regularly, and my entire visual system remains relaxed.

As I read I breathe evenly, blink regularly, and my entire visual system remains relaxed.

The black print appears in clear contrast to the glowing whiteness, and I see clearly as I read.

The black print appears in clear contrast to the glowing whiteness, and I see clearly as I read.

The black print appears in clear contrast to the glowing whiteness, and I see clearly as I read.

The black print appears in clear contrast to the glowing whiteness, and I see clearly as I read.

The black print appears in clear contrast to the glowing whiteness, and I see clearly as I read.

The black print appears in clear contrast to the glowing whiteness, and I see clearly as I read.

The black print appears in clear contrast to the glowing whiteness, and I see clearly as I read.

The black print appears in clear contrast to the glowing whiteness, and I see clearly as I read.

My youthful, revitalized lenses are so flexible that they effortlessly adjust for clear vision close up.

My youthful, revitalized lenses are so flexible that they effortlessly adjust for clear vision close up.

My youthful, revitalized lenses are so flexible that they effortlessly adjust for clear vision close up.

My youthful, revitalized lenses are so flexible that they effortlessly adjust for clear vision close up.

My youthful, revitalized lenses are so flexible that they effortlessly adjust for clear vision close up.

My youthful, revitalized lenses are so flexible that they effortlessly adjust for clear vision close up.

My youthful, revitalized lenses are so flexible that they effortlessly adjust for clear vision close up.

My youthful, revitalized lenses are so flexible that they effortlessly adjust for clear vision close up.

I slide my eyes under the lines of print, aware of the whiteness, and the black print is clear in contrast.

I slide my eyes under the lines of print, aware of the whiteness, and the black print is clear in contrast.

I slide my eyes under the lines of print, aware of the whiteness, and the black print is clear in contrast.

I slide my eyes under the lines of print, aware of the whiteness, and the black print is clear in contrast.

I slide my eyes under the lines of print, aware of the whiteness, and the black print is clear in contrast.

I slide my eyes under the lines of print, aware of the whiteness, and the black print is clear in contrast.

I slide my eyes under the lines of print, aware of the whiteness, and the black print is clear in contrast.

I slide my eyes under the lines of print, aware of the whiteness, and the black print is clear in contrast.

My visual system is relaxed, my lenses are flexible, and I see clearly up close.

My visual system is relaxed, my lenses are flexible, and I see clearly up close.

My visual system is relaxed, my lenses are flexible, and I see clearly up close.

My visual system is relaxed, my lenses are flexible, and I see clearly up close.

My visual system is relaxed, my lenses are flexible, and I see clearly up close.

My visual system is relaxed, my lenses are flexible, and I see clearly up close.

My visual system is relaxed, my lenses are flexible, and I see clearly up close.

My visual system is relaxed, my lenses are flexible, and I see clearly up close.

Remain palming as long as you like, then count yourself up into full alertness, feeling rested, refreshed, and confident of your ability to see clearly at nearpoint.

In essence, that's it! By the end of this fourth week your lenses should be fully rejuvenated and you should once again be able to read without glasses. Having said this, let me point out that the timing here is based on an average. We are all a little different, so don't be overly concerned if you haven't yet completely achieved your goal. If there is obviously some work left to be done, get out your pendulum so you can pinpoint just where to concentrate further efforts.

The pendulum, as you'll remember from Chapter 5, will provide you with a direct line of communication to your subconscious. Your inner mind will tell you where you need more work. Even if you have attained clear reading vision now, you may want to use the pendulum to pick up clues on how to maintain this skill.

Take out your pendulum and reestablish the directional swings that will signify "yes," "no", and "I don't know." Then, as a warmup, ask yourself some simple yes-and-no questions that you already know the answers to, such as your birth date, age, and favorite color. Once warmed up, ask the following questions one at a time. Be patient as you wait for the answers. Your subconscious may need a little time to consider each possibility.

1. Are my lenses receiving enough circulation? If you get a no answer, proceed on with these supplementary questions:
    a. Do I need more hypnotic suggestions for an increase of circulation to my lenses?
    b. Do I need more massage to increase the circulation into my lenses?
    c. Do I need more physical exercise in order to increase the circulation into my lenses?
2. Are my lenses receiving enough nutrients? If you get a no answer to this, continue on with the following:
    a. Is the lack of nutrients due to poor circulation?
    b. Do I need to improve my diet in order for my lenses to receive more nutrients?
3. Do I need more practice with the fusion string?
4. Do I need more practice with the Near and Far charts?
5. Do I need more practice with the reading exercises?

Your subconscious will supply the answers you need. If there are any other factors in your life-style, such as smoking, that you think might influence your sight, ask about those too. Once you have the information you need, you'll be able to go back to the parts of the program that apply and repeat them.

Once you have achieved the success you desire, use bits and pieces of the program that are your favorites as maintenance. Even though I stress this, I must admit that some of my clients have sustained their nearpoint reading ability for several years without any continued work at all. Most, however, just continue on with the enjoyable massages and suggestions whether they need it or not. They add suggestions for enhancing other aspects of their lives as well. Once you've activated the healing power of your mind, you can apply it to any mental or physical concern. Use it freely, it belongs to you. You have nothing at all to lose and a life of accomplishment and positive well-being to gain. Enjoy!

The Hyperopia Program

If you have hyperopia, the type of farsightedness that develops early in life, and you've mastered the art of hypnotizing yourself, then you can expect a great deal of positive changes in your vision over the next eight weeks. Because hyperopes by nature tend to be more outwardly rather than inwardly focused, the process of gaining the inward focus required for both hypnosis and vision work can sometimes be slow in coming. So don't rush on with the program until you feel you relax well into the hypnotic state and are able really to feel the imagined sensations of body breathing, moving down, and being unable to open your eyes. Take your time and enjoy this inward focusing of your attention.

If you'll recall, in Chapter 3 I said that this type of farsightedness occurs when the eyeball is too short from front to back. There is most likely accompanying inflexibility in the lens as well, as there is in presbyopia, but in hyperopia, the shape of the eye is as important as it is for its polar opposite, myopia. The recti extraocular muscles that stretch from front to back on the eye are so tight that the eye is somewhat flattened and the incoming image is focused behind the retina, whereas in myopia the oblique muscles that band the eye cause an elongation of the eye so that the image falls in front of the retina.

We all begin life a little hyperopic because the eyes aren't finished growing and developing when we are born. By the time they start school, quite a few children still haven't attained the full length of their eyes and flexibility of their lenses. Only recently has this been recognized as a cause of many reading problems. These children have no difficulty reading the blackboard, but when reading material close up they experience eye strain. This manifests in headaches, visual fatigue, an inability to focus attention for long on nearpoint work, and even behavioral problems. Fortunately, many teachers are now aware of these signs and refer children to eye doctors. A simple reading lens for a few years can serve these youngsters well until their eyes finish growing. If the problem is not attended to, however, so much tension is created trying to force vision that the recti muscles go into cramped spasm and continue to keep the eyeball shortened. In addition to this, personality and emotional factors tend to accompany hyperopia. Again, they are quite the opposite of those seen in myopes. There are always exceptions, but see if you fit into the hyperopic tendencies.

I've already mentioned that hyperopes tend to be outwardly directed rather than inwardly so. Are you more extroverted rather than introverted? More sports oriented as opposed to sedentary? Does your posture tend to be somewhat stiff, perhaps with the back of your neck so straight and tight that it actually interferes with your ability to turn your head easily from side to side? Do you hold your chest high and expanded? Chances are you are a good visualizer yet are also very much aware of everything around you. Do your eyes feel fatigued if you read for a long time? Do you have other difficulties in reading? Do you suffer from headaches? Crossed eyes?

Some of these tendencies may reflect an underlying emotional predisposition. Dr. Charles Kelley of the Radix Institute is responsible for the most insightful studies of the emotional factors that pertain to visual dysfunctions, myopia and hyperopia in particular. Whereas he found myopes to be blocking emotions of fear, he determined hyperopes to have deep-seated feelings of anger. This is something to consider within yourself, especially if you haven't made as much progress as you want by the end of the program. The chances are good that you've actually worked out this inner attitude through growing and maturing, and the subconscious visual tension established early in your life will respond readily to retraining. But if the muscles don't let go so that your eyes can assume an optimal shape, you'll want to look deeper into the emotional issues. By the use of your pendulum and Chapter 12, "Regression," you can discover what is holding you back and resolve it. Hypnosis is a gentle yet thorough technique for identifying emotional memories and then becoming liberated from them.

A good example of recovery from severe hyperopia is Lynn, a middle-age woman whose glasses magnified her eyes so much that she looked like a startled owl. Her progress was not coming along well until I regressed her. She remembered that her mother was constantly angry with her because she couldn't remember to put her toys away, even though she was only three. She, in turn, was furious with her mother but was afraid to lash back because such behavior was always punished by being locked in a dark closet. So she learned to block her anger, but it manifested itself in her eyesight. These memories were very liberating for Lynn. Her sight improved to the point where glasses could be prescribed that didn't make her eyes seem so prominent. Even more important, she was able to remember positive as well as negative things about her mother, which gave her much peace of mind.

The basic program lasts eight weeks and is almost a mirror image of the myopia program. This book would be too bulky if I rewrote every session to perfectly match each visual condition. The suggestions are lengthy and very carefully worked out, the closest I could come to duplicating those I use with my everyday clients. You'll primarily use the scripts provided for myopia and replace the key terms and phrases with ones that apply for you.

For example, you'll suggest that your eyeballs become longer as opposed to shorter. You will also have one session that is drawn from the presbyopia program. As you progress, be sure to read everything in Chapter 6, all the introductory material as well as the sessions themselves. That chapter is the model upon which all the others are based, and it contains vital information and instructions that apply to all types of vision. Just remember to keep in mind the ways in which you differ from those with myopia. Also, take time to study the illustration comparing the normal, myopic, and hyperopic eyes (see page 23). Many of your suggestions and visualizations will center on the physical changes that must take place in your eyes so that they come to conform to the optimal shape.

WEEK ONE

Polar opposite that you might be to a myope, the suggestions for this first week will still be very similar because you are dealing primarily with your belief system. All else will follow naturally once your inner mind is convinced of its ability to effect change. You will, however, be changing some key words and phrases. Once you have read all the introductory information, you will go on to make changes in the myopia script beginning on page 59 so that your particular eye shape, muscles, and desired distance of clear focus will be addressed properly. I recommend that you photocopy the suggestions for myopia and then write in the changes on your copy before tape-recording the session.

First, go through the script looking for references to *ciliary* and *oblique* muscles (the word *ciliary* appears six times, *oblique* three). They don't apply to your condition, so you will eliminate them, and in their place you will substitute *lenses* and *recti*. For example, the eighth sentence is the first to mention ciliary and oblique muscles. It reads *"Your ciliary and oblique extraocular muscles are relaxing more and more."* You will change this sentence to read *"Your lenses and recti extraocular muscles are relaxing more and more."* Make similar alterations throughout the script.

Next you will need to change the references to the desired shape of the eye from *rounder* and its variations *round* and *rounding* to *longer, long,* or *elongating.* This first occurs in the ninth sentence. It reads *"They are relaxing so much that your lenses and eyeballs are free to come into a rounder shape."* You will change this sentence so that it reads *"They are relaxing so much that your lenses and eyeballs are free to come into a longer shape."* There are five of these references.

Three times you will see the phrase *in the distance*. Change it to *up close*. Some people prefer to say *at nearpoint*. Use a phrase that sounds good to you.

There are also three references to *positive changes that will bring you clear vision at all distances*. You need to add one important key word to this so it reads *positive changes that will bring you clear and* comfortable *vision at all distances*. Hyperopia tends to involve some uncomfortable eye strain, so you definitely want to transform that into comfortable as well as clear vision.

Toward the end of the suggestions, on page 61, there is an important sentence that needs a lot of changes. For myopes it reads *"From now on, when you look into the distance your ciliary and oblique muscles will relax, and you will see more clearly."* Change it so that it reads *"From now on, when you focus at nearpoint your recti muscles will relax and your ciliary muscles will pull your flexible lenses into a flatter, longer, more concave shape, and you will see more clearly."*

Those are the only changes you will have to make in the suggestions this week. Don't forget to make changes in the minisessions as well (page 63). The words *ciliary, oblique,* and *into the distance* appear only once, and the word *shorter* should be changed to *longer*.

WEEK TWO

This is even easier than last week. Read over pages 64 to 75. You'll enjoy the same benefits of massage reflected in your vision as well as your general sense of well-being, and the script changes are minimal. There are none in the first session. In the second, simply change *oblique* to *recti* and again take out references to *ciliary muscles* and substitute *lenses*. (Both words appear only three times.) The words *in the distance* and *into the distance,* which both appear once, should be changed to *at all distances*. The only major change appears on page 73. There are directions for cupping your hands and making rounding and flattening movements. Your directions will be just the reverse of those for the myopes. For example, the text now reads *"Continue on this way, concentrating on the rounding movement rather than the flattening movement. Each time you round your hands, your eyes also become rounder and shorter from front to back.*" You will substitute the following: "*Continue on this way, concentrating on the flattening movement rather than the rounding movement. Each time you flatten your hands, your eyes also become elongated from front to back.*" Continue making the same changes in the sentences that follow directly. All the rest of your interconnected muscles and your visual system will respond as needed to the same suggestions. Massage is wonderful, enjoy!

WEEK THREE

Once again there are just a few word changes to be made so that this week is as appropriate for you as for myopes. As you'll see when you read through pages 75 to 85, there are three parts to the sessions. The first, long swings, is done with your vision directed out into the distance. This will be fine for you as well, since the visual loosening accomplished through this exercise applies to all eyes. Omit the one reference to the *ciliary muscles* altogether. Change *oblique* to *recti* and *rounder* to *longer. Oblique* appears just once, *rounder* twice. And change the phrase "*you see more clearly in the distance*" to "*you see clearly at all distances*" both times it appears. For example, toward the bottom of page 79 there is a sentence that reads "*Muscles relaxed, eyes rounder, you see more clearly in the distance.*" You will change it to read "*Muscles relaxed, eyes longer, you see more clearly at all distances.*"

In the second section, sunning, all you'll need to do is take out the three references to *ciliary muscles* altogether, change three references to *oblique* to *recti*, and the four times the words *round, rounder,* or *rounding* appear, change them to *longer* and *lengthening.*

In the third phase, short swings, there are no key word changes but you'll be changing the size and distance of the imagined white card. You want to stimulate your near vision, so instead of a three-by-five card out in the distance, you will imagine a much smaller and closer card. Let yours be a one-by-two card approximately a foot in front of you. You will still be actually moving your head a bit along with the visualization. The swinging movement of your head will be very small but very effective. One of Dr. Bates's discoveries was the smaller the swing, the greater the relaxation. At the same time that your recti muscles will be relaxing, you also want to encourage your lenses to contract into the flatter, more concave shape for near vision, so include a suggestion for that that reads "As you swing, your eyes lengthen and your ciliary muscles pull your lenses into a flatter, more convex shape, and you see clearly up close."

WEEK FOUR

This week you will adapt the two visualizations given in the myopia chapter (pages 85–93) to your own special needs. The first is a series of scenes in nature. Originally I had hyperopes imagine that they were watching these scenes on a close tiny television screen. If you find this idea appealing, use the script that is supplied. However, many hyperopes felt cheated that they didn't get to feel as if they were in the scene. If you find you feel the same way, some simple adjustments to the script will supply you with opportunities to utilize your nearpoint mental vision. Have every animal come in to you and examine them up close. Imagine walking up to objects on the ship and foliage on the land and seeing the details clearly. If it doesn't present an undesirable reminder of the real world, imagine you are wearing a watch that you bring very close to your face as you check the time. You can also imagine that you are carrying a magazine or a book with you on this journey which you occasionally take time out to read. If you do this, study a particular page of a real magazine beforehand so that you will know what you're looking at.

Change the minisession suggestions just as you have been doing all along.

The second visualization involves seeing and feeling the physiological changes in your eyes and then imagining golden healing energy transforming your eyes and visual system. You won't have to make any changes during the energy visualization, but the ones you'll need in the first half are more extensive than usual. For this reason I'll fully detail them for you.

You will begin making changes with the fifth sentence on page 91. Alter it to read "*As your lenses and recti muscles relax, your eyes have room to stretch into a more elongated shape."* Change the next sentence to read *"Longer from front to back than before."*

A few sentences later there is one that reads *"See those oblique extraocular muscles around your eyes."* Change this to *"See those recti extraocular muscles that stretch from the front to the back of your eyes."* Leave the next sentence the way it is, but change the following one to read *"See and feel the constricted shortness in your eyeballs caused by these tight recti muscles."*

As you continue, change *oblique* to *recti* and *short* to *long.* When you see *round out,* change it to *lengthen.*

When you reach the section that begins *"Now imagine a pair of healing hands coming into this picture,"* eliminate that whole segment up to *"Let the image fade away . . ."* In its place you will visualize a massage to your lenses. Let it read as follows: *"Now let the healing hands move on to your lenses. First see them as round and stiff. As the healing hands massage your lenses, they immediately begin to look and feel softer. The hands are massaging circulation, relaxation, and flexibility into your lenses. Feel your lenses relax and soften as the hands massage them into a more concave shape. Your lenses are flexible, and they can now adapt to the concave shape for clear nearpoint vision. See and feel your lenses being massaged, softened, relaxed. Your ciliary muscles can easily pull your flexible lenses into the concave shape for clear nearpoint vision. See your lenses in a relaxed concave shape. . . ."* Now continue as written except for changing *oblique* to *recti* in the next sentence.

In the myopia introduction to this week, you will notice that I suggest reversing the order of the visualizations if you are going to go to sleep after the evening session. This applies to you as well.

WEEK FIVE

Once again you will change *oblique* to *recti* (it appears five times), and the three references to the distance at which you see clearly (pages 93–99). Leave in references to your ciliary muscles. This will reinforce their continued proper functioning. And, instead of practicing the visual skills laid out in the session using the room or scenery around you, you will use magazine or calendar pictures.

The best ones to use are those that include both a lot of color and detail as well as some print to read. Scenic calendars are perfect for this. When you begin the exercise, hold the picture close enough so that some of the finest details are difficult for you to see. As the session goes on you'll find your near vision improving beautifully. As you're edging and scanning the pictures, let your nose lead. It's as if you have a pencil attached to the end of your nose. Be sure to read the introductory material carefully.

WEEK SIX

This week you'll use the sixth week of the myopia program for your first full session and the seventh week for your second session. The first is called string fusion. Read through pages 99–107. You'll find that you have good fusion ability when looking out to the end of the fusion string. You want to develop that same ease of focus at the end of the string closest to you. If you find that you have a lot of difficulty with the two closest knots, add extra ones so that your eyes have a chance to improve in smaller increments. You will also be starting the exercise focused on the farthest knot and ending it on the closest one, both in the imaginary fusing and the actual one.

The changes you will be making in the myopia script will include both the reversal of the order of the knots as well as the usual ones for eye shape and lens adjustment. By renaming your knots, you won't have to change much wording in the directions. Let your first knot be the one farthest away from you. The fourth knot for myopes will be your second knot, and so on. You'll begin doing this with the first direction, *"Imagine focusing on the knot closest to you"* (see page 103). Change that to *"Imagine focusing on the knot farthest away from you."* The next line reads *"Clearly see the short ghost strings coming into it and the long ones extending out from it in a V shape."* Change this to read *"Clearly see the long strings coming in toward you in the shape of an inverted V."* Follow this same procedure as you continue.

Suggestions for the functioning of your eyes begin on page 103, just before imagining seeing the knotted string and its optical illusion ghost strings with the sentence that reads *"Your ciliary and oblique muscles relax as you stretch your vision into the distance, and you see clearly.* " This should read *"Your recti muscles relax and your ciliary muscles pull your flexible lenses into a concave shape as you look up close, and you see clearly."* You'll find four opportunities to make this change throughout the script.

For your minisessions this week, use the one for the sixth week of myopia (see page 107), making your usual changes.

For your second full session, move on to the seventh week of the myopia program (pages 107–115), and adapt it by reversing everything. You will begin looking at the distant letters on the far chart, and when you pull your gaze in, your *recti* muscles will relax, your eyes will *elongate,* and your *ciliary muscles* will pull your lenses into the *flatter, more concave* shape for clear *nearpoint* vision. You can leave in the references to your ciliary and oblique muscles relaxing when you look into the distance. They already do that, but it's good reinforcement to keep it up. Hold the Near Chart close enough in the beginning so that the letters aren't quite clear, so that you'll experience your vision improving during the session.

So that you'll fully understand how to make changes in the chart work, I'll rewrite instructions covering the first two letters for you. It begins with imagining the letter *F.* Your script will read "Now imagine that you are looking at a white card in your hand with the black letter *F* on it. But let the *F* appear a little blurry and a little gray instead of dark black. Now imagine looking out into the distance to a white piece of paper with an *F* on it. This one is very clear, and there is a sharp contrast between the white background and the dark, black *F.* Study the *F,* noting that it is made up of three black lines and that it stands out clearly against the white. As you do this the optic center of your brain is memorizing the *F.* In a moment it will direct your eyes to function so well that the near *F* will seem just as close as the distant one. It does that now as you imagine looking in to the near *F.* Now you see it clearly, clear black lines against the white background. Your brain directed your ciliary muscles to pull your flexible lenses into the concave shape for nearpoint vision, and the image became clear. Your brain and your eyes are capable of making these adjustments so you see clearly up close. . . . Now replace the *F* with an *O,* but let it seem closer, so as the *F* was in the beginning, now the *O* is a little gray and blurry. Imagine looking out at the white paper in the distance and seeing a clear, black *O*. Study its shape and be aware of the contrast between the black and the white. Your brain is memorizing this *O* and will direct your eyes to see it clearly at nearpoint. Imagine looking in to the close *O* and now seeing it perfectly clearly. Your eyes and brain are capable of making the necessary adjustments so that you see clearly up close. . . ."

Follow this example and change all of the imagined and real chart instructions in the same way.

WEEK SEVEN

This week you practice reading at nearpoint. You'll use the scripts for the fourth week of the *presbyopia* program (see pages 161–171). The only change is to include suggestions for your *recti* muscles relaxing and your eyes *elongating*. Add them whenever you see suggestions for the flexibility of your lenses. For example, after the second sentence, *"My lenses are youthful and flexible,"* add *"My recti muscles are relaxing and my eyes elongating."* You'll make this change three more times in the first script and three times in all in the second script. Your eyes are primed to be able to read up close now, and these exercises will give your eyes a chance to work with their new skills.

WEEK EIGHT

The sessions this week are overall reviews of everything you've done so far (see pages 116–128). Just make all the same changes that you did before, and add the reading from each of the sessions for your week seven to the scripts given for myopia. Read through both scripts once during both sessions. If you haven't made all the progress you'd hoped for, go through the procedure with the pendulum in the same way you have for the sessions, changing the key words. Hopefully you won't need this last step, and congratulations are definitely in order. If there's still more to be done, persevere!

The Astigmatism Program

If you're astigmatic, this program will enable you to balance the muscular pull on your corneas and allow them to smooth out. The distorted, overlapping images you have been experiencing will relax into clear, distinct ones. The program laid out in this chapter is a four-week one designed for those of you who have astigmatism as your only visual problem. However, the odds are that your astigmatism occurs in conjunction with some other visual dysfunction, most likely myopia or hyperopia. For those of you in this majority, you will be adding the specific suggestions for astigmatism to the program for your more predominant problem, which will probably be an eight-week program.

As you'll see when you get into the program, the core of it is based on the myopia program. In addition to making changes in the scripts, be sure to read the entire myopia chapter (Chapter 6) thoroughly. You may also want to review the material about astigmatism in Chapter 3, "Why We Don't See Clearly." Both chapters contain information that will enable you to fully understand the nature of the changes you want to achieve.

The easiest way to make your script changes is to photocopy the original material and make changes on your copy before tape-recording it. If you are not myopic, don't be overly concerned with eliminating every reference to this condition. Do the best you can to remove what doesn't specifically apply to you, but be aware that these references won't have a negative impact on your sight if they are left in. They'll just serve as reinforcements of your already good vision.

Contrary to the traditional optometric belief, astigmatism is very fluid and very amenable to improvement. All it takes is a poor night's sleep or other stress to create astigmatism. Conversely, it will smooth out on its own once the stress is removed, provided glasses don't lock it into the visual system. Most eye doctors may chuckle at you, but they are easily persuaded to reduce the correction for astigmatism in your glasses by 50 percent. If not too much astigmatism is apparent, they'll cooperate and take out all of the correction. Your eyes will respond much more quickly to the program if you have no correction for astigmatism at all. However, do not have your prescription reduced to the point where you can no longer drive safely.

If you had an emotional background of reacting to events with the confusion that so often creates astigmatism, you have most likely outgrown it. However, that same habitual response pattern is still locked in your visual system. You'll not only be relaxing your recti muscles into alignment and smoothing out your corneas, but you'll also be reeducating the optic center of your brain to send out a new set of signals as you use your eyes.

Tom, a young stockbroker, had mild myopia accompanied by moderate astigmatism. His father was a career army officer, so the family moved often as Tom was growing up. During regression he remembered a number of instances when he felt lost and lonely in new towns and schools. Once he understood at the subconscious level that he was no longer in danger of being a lost little boy, both of his conditions improved dramatically. The myopia was simply due to excessive reading by a shy youngster. In addition to his other exercises, Tom particularly enjoyed the long swings, which are wonderful for smoothing out astigmatism. He did them to soft background music every day for fifteen minutes. By the end of eight weeks he had no need for his glasses except for night driving.

In rare instances astigmatism forms in the lens or the retina instead of the cornea. If your eye doctor has informed you that you are one of this minority, simply suggest during the hypnotic induction that the affected area is where the balancing and smoothing is occurring. We don't know how these kinds of astigmatism come about, but I have worked with a few and they responded to Hypno-Vision.

WEEK ONE

In Chapter 3 I mentioned that quite a few astigmatics have notice-ably lopsided posture with more tension on one side than on the other. If you have looked in a mirror and found this to be true in your case, let me again emphasize the value of certain forms of exercise, bodywork, and massage. The massage that will be part of your program is wonderful for astigmatism, but more aligning of the whole body is often necessary. All types of whole-body massage will have a profound impact on your body. Yoga is a gentle form of exercise that will straighten and balance you. The Feldenkrais method (there are teachers in nearly every major city as well as books on the subject) is another method of gentle movement that has phenomenal physical benefits. Find out what is available near you, and do your whole body as well as your eyes a favor.

In this first week, just as in the rest of the program, those of you who have another visual problem, say myopia, will simply add the additional suggestions given below to your core program. If you have astigmatism alone, your first full session each day this week will use the corresponding one for the first week of the myopia program (see page 59). To it you will add and remove a few key words. Throughout the script you will see occasional references to *ciliary and oblique extraocular muscles*. If you are not myopic, remove *oblique* and replace it with *recti*. If you are myopic *and* astigmatic, on the other hand, you would say *oblique and recti extraocular muscles*. When you see mention of *extraocular muscles* without specific ones men-tioned leave the suggestion alone, as it reinforces a positive, general relaxing and balancing of all your eye muscles.

You will also see the term *round* or *rounder* used in conjunction with eyeball and lens shape. These terms will change or be ex-panded upon depending upon your needs. For example, the first sentence you will alter (on page 59) reads, *"They are relaxing so much that your lenses and eyeballs are free to come into a rounder shape."* If you are only astigmatic you will change it to read *"They are relaxing so much that your corneas are free to smooth out."* If you are myopic as well as astigmatic, expand the suggestion so that it reads *"They are relaxing so much that your lenses and eyeballs are free to come into a rounder shape, and your corneas are free to smooth out."* If, on the other hand, you are hyperopic and astigmatic, the sentence will read *"They are relaxing so much that your eyeballs are free to come into a more elongated shape, and your corneas are free to smooth out."*

You will also find suggestions for clear distance vision. You, of course, want to make the emphasis on clear vision at *all* distances.

In addition to these changes, there is a one-sentence suggestion that will add special encouragement to your visual system to smooth out your astigmatism. Three times during the script, at points that feel appropriate to you, insert the following: *"My recti muscles are relaxed, aligned, and balanced, and my corneas are smooth."*

The script for your minisessions this week will be the same as the one for myopia (see page 63), with the same changes you made for the full session. Also, add the suggestion given above, once.

Your second full session for this week will be based on the second session of week four of the myopia program (see pages 91–93). This is a series of visualizations that will activate the healing power within your subconscious mind. As you remove the suggestions that apply to myopia detailed above, insert ones for first seeing a tight, imbalanced pull of your recti muscles and a warping of your cornea. As the massage takes place you will see and feel the recti muscles relaxing, balancing, and aligning and the cornea smoothing out. For example, when the healing hands first come into the picture, your suggestions should read as follows: *"See them kneading and massaging your imbalanced recti muscles. As you see the muscles respond to this healing touch and relax, feel the relaxation as well. As the muscles relax they come into perfect, balanced alignment, and your corneas are free to smooth out. See your corneas smoothing out. It feels so good to have those muscles massaged, and as they relax your corneas smooth out. . . ."* Keep seeing, feeling, and affirming these changes instead of those for myopia. Don't be surprised if these sessions this first week bring about a noticeable improvement in your vision.

WEEK TWO

During your second week you'll enjoy the physical massage, as opposed to the mental healing one, for your first full session. For it you will use the first session of the second week of the myopia program (see pages 64–68). The only change is to add *balancing and aligning* whenever there is a reference to your eye muscles *relaxing*. It is likely that you will find more tension on one side of your neck than the other, so give yourself a little extra massaging attention where you feel you need it. Be aware of your vision when you finish the massaging, as your images will be sharp and clear.

Your minisessions this week are drawn from the fifth week of the myopia program (see page 99). Again, instead of the reference to your *ciliary* and *oblique* muscles, include references to your *recti* muscles relaxing, aligning, and balancing and your corneas smoothing out.

The second session will also utilize the one for the fifth week of the myopia program (see pages 93–99) and will teach your eyes to relax and move smoothly as you use them. This pleasant and relaxing little exercise will return relaxed, spontaneous movement to your vision as your eyes have a chance to practice the new skills they are learning. Instead of the specifics pertaining to myopia, you will keep affirming that your recti muscles are relaxed, aligned, and balanced, and that they all work together as a coordinated team. Affirm also that your corneas are smooth and you see clearly at all distances. You'll find the portion of the exercise called edging will have a particularly beneficial effect on your vision.

WEEK THREE

Your third week will continue the smoothing and balancing process with a combination of relaxing movement and specific focusing of your eyes through the improved balance and alignment of your recti muscles. For your first session follow the script for the third week of the myopia program (see pages 75–85), which covers relaxing exercises known as long swings, sunning, and short swings. Make the same alterations for the relaxing, balancing, and aligning of your recti muscles and the smoothing of your corneas that you have been making so far. I've seen many eyes smooth out beautifully with this session alone, so you can expect even better results because you've done so much preliminary work already.

The minisessions for this week will combine suggestions to reinforce both full sessions. After rapidly inducing your hypnotic state, you will affirm the following:

o

"My eyes are wonderfully relaxed and energized. . . . Every time I swing, sun, and visualize my sight improves. . . . My recti muscles are relaxed, balanced, and aligned. . . . My corneas are smooth. . . . My eyes work as a relaxed and perfectly coordinated team. . . . I see clearly at all distances. . . . My eyes balance as I scan for detail, and I see clearly at all distances. . . . My eyes are balanced and aligned, and my shoulders, neck, head, and facial muscles relax as my eyes balance and align. . . . I am ready for clear vision. I deserve clear vision. I am confident my vision is improving."

o

For your second session use the script for week six of the myopia program, the string fusion exercise (see pages 99–107). This one really puts your new skills to work. Make those same substitutions of your relaxed, balanced, and aligned recti muscles for the ones that apply to myopia. Optometrists who use this exercise often find that it actually causes more astigmatism. It will have quite the opposite effect for you, because your eyes and visual system will be constantly reminded to relax as you work with them.

WEEK FOUR

This final phase is an all-encompassing refresher week that puts shortened versions of everything you've done so far into one session that you will do twice a day. It will be similar to the eighth week for myopes (see pages 116–128), but, of course, you don't have nearly as much material to cover. Your session will include the introductory and summing-up suggestions as well as the sections on shoulder/neck/head massage (session one of myopia), sunning and swinging (session one of myopia), string fusion (session one of myopia), healing and energy visualization (session two of myopia), and edging and scanning (session two of myopia). You will be leaving out the acupressure massage and the chart work. Remove the specific suggestions for myopia about shape of the eyes and relaxation of the lenses and ciliary muscles, and substitute ones for the relaxing, balancing, and aligning of your recti muscles and the smoothing out of your corneas. If the session runs too long, break it down into two, like those for myopia.

In between your full sessions, use the following suggestions for your minisessions:

o

"My vision is relaxed, spontaneous, and clear. . . . I see clearly at all distances. . . . My recti muscles are relaxed, balanced, and aligned. . . . My corneas are smooth. . . . I see clear, distinct images. . . . My eyes function in perfect relaxed alignment and I see clearly. . . . My neck and shoulder muscles are relaxed, balanced, and aligned. . . . The optic center of my brain directs my eyes to see clearly, and it interprets the images sent to it as clear. . . . I am absolutely confident of the clarity of my vision. . . . I see clearly."

o

Astigmatism responds so well to the techniques in the HypnoVision program that you will probably see vast improvement during this four-week period. If you don't improve as much as you wished, follow the directions for pendulum use on pages 127–128.

10

Other Vision Problems

The basics of the HypnoVision program can be applied successfully to any visual problem. In this chapter you'll find instructions for choosing and tailoring the scripts so they will be effective for you. Besides making the changes within the scripts, be sure to read the introductory material in the chapters you are referred to. If your condition is so rare that it is not included in this section, you can create your own script changes. Ask your eye doctor or read up on the specifics of your problem and use them to build your suggestions.

Before embarking on your program, be sure to read all of the introductory material for the myopia program (Chapter 6). It is the core of the book and contains vital directions and information for all types of vision. Also, whenever your sessions are based on scripts from the myopia program, be sure to read the preliminary material that accompanies each of them. Likewise, if you are directed to draw from the presbyopia program (Chapter 7), study that introductory material as well.

In addition to making the script changes detailed in this chapter, you can add suggestions that have a special meaning for you. If you do this, be sure to use the same positive phrasing style that I have used. Never use negatives because your subconscious tends to omit them. For example, "The circulation into my eyes is not as constricted as before" would be a negative suggestion. Your subconscious would focus on the idea of your circulation being restricted. A positive suggestion would be "The circulation into my eyes is more open than before." This latter suggestion is positive, but it can be improved. Always make suggestions as strong as possible. "The circulation into my eyes is open" would be simpler and better. The easiest way to make the necessary script changes is to photocopy the suggestions and make changes on your copy before tape-recording.

If You Wear Bifocals or Trifocals

If you wear bifocals or trifocals, your eight-week program will draw scripts from the myopia, presbyopia, and hyperopia programs. This way you will regain clear vision at all distances. Most people needed just reading glasses before a correction for distance vision was also added. Many myopes retain their ability to focus clearly at near-point despite the aging process. But if you were nearsighted before you also needed a reading lens, this chapter is for you too. If you have been wearing a correction for near, far, and even middle distances for more than a few years, you may need to be patient and stay with the program longer than the allotted eight weeks. But this is better news than I could have given you before I integrated hypnosis into vision work. While a weakened prescription was the only realistic expectation in the past, with the HypnoVision approach I have seen a number of clients improve their vision so much that they were able to discard reading glasses as well as their distance lenses.

WEEK ONE

Your first session of each day this week will address your distance vision. You'll use the script for week one of the myopia program (see pages 57–62). For your minisessions, use the ones for the myopia program (see page 63) but add suggestions from the presbyopia session about the circulation in and flexibility of your lenses (see page 136). Your second full session will move on to your near vision, and you'll use the script for week one of the presbyopia program (see pages 132–136).

WEEK TWO

This week you'll be continuing to relax your eye muscles and send circulation to your lenses through a different massage during each of your two sessions. You will follow almost same format that you did last week. For your first session use the first session from week two of the myopia program (see pages 64–68). For your minisessions again include suggestions for the flexibility of your lenses in with those given for myopia. For your second session, use the *second* session for week two of the presbyopia program (see pages 142–146).

WEEK THREE

This week you'll do the same set of exercises in each session, but one will contain suggestions for your distance vision and the other for your near vision. For the morning session, use the script for week three of the myopia program (see pages 75–85). Your second full session will use the script for week three of the hyperopia program (see pages 178–179). However, the hyperopia scripts are all revised versions of the myopia scripts. This means that your hyperopia script will be your rewrite of the one you used for myopia, as will be the hyperopia scripts you'll use in weeks four and five. For your minisession combine the suggestions for clear close and distance vision that you find for this week in the myopia and hyperopia sessions. As usual, combine suggestions for your minisessions.

WEEK FOUR

This is an enjoyable week made up of two separate visualizations. The first is one of beautiful scenes in nature. You'll do it exactly as presented in the first session of week four of the myopia program (see pages 85–89). Use the minisession from the myopia program (page 90) with the usual addition of suggestions for flexibility of your lenses. For your second session you'll use the second session for week four of the hyperopia program (see pages 179–180).

WEEK FIVE

As in week three, now you will again do the same session twice, once for your distance vision and once for your near vision. Your first session will be the same as week five of the myopia program (see pages 93–99). Make the usual changes regarding the flexibility of your lenses in the myopia minisession (page 99). Your second session will be the same as week five of the hyperopia program (see page 180).

WEEK SIX

This week you will develop your fusion and accommodation skills. In the early session you'll work on fusion, using the session from week six of the myopia program (see pages 99–106). Combine the minisession suggestions for myopia (page 107) and presbyopia (page 136) into one that reinforces your near and distance vision. Your second session will concentrate on accommodation, and you'll use the script for the second session of week three of the presbyopia session (see pages 153–160).

WEEK SEVEN

This week focuses on the development of your nearpoint reading ability. You will follow the exact script for week four of the presbyopia program (see pages 161–166), including the minisession. You'll find your near vision improves dramatically during this week.

WEEK EIGHT

This week is a review of everything you've done. In the first session use the script for the first session of week eight of the myopia program (see pages 116–121). In it include the reading from week four of the presbyopia program (see pages 161–166). However, just read each of the scripts once. Use the myopia minisessions (page 121) with additions from week four of presbyopia (page 166). For the second session use the script for the second session of week eight of the hyperopia program (see page 183), again including the texts for both presbyopia reading exercises.

Hopefully, all that's in order after this week is hearty congratulations. If after these eight weeks you haven't improved both your near and distance vision as much as you wanted, find out what else you need to do through the use of the pendulum. Use the questions from both the myopia section (pages 127–128) and the presbyopia section (page 172).

Strabismus

If you have an eye or eyes that turn in or out, you have what's called *strabismus.* It is caused by an imbalanced pull of the recti muscles. One is very tight and pulls the eye out of alignment. Two very different images are perceived by the brain, so one is usually shut off entirely. This results in a lack of depth perception in addition to the cosmetic problem of appearance. In some cases the nerves in the retina also shut down, and the result is *amblyopia,* or lazy-eye blindness. You know you have this condition if you see little or nothing with the turned eye when you close the good one. If this is the case for you, you will first deal with that problem in the section on amblyopia that follows (see page 202) before you work with this one for strabismus.

Most people with strabismus also have either hyperopia or myopia as well. If you have a companion condition, you will be attending to it while you also work on straightening your eyes. If the turning of an eye is your only problem, your program will be shorter. Either way you need one extra piece of equipment, an eye patch. You will be using both eyes together part of the time but will be patching your good eye the rest of the time.

The causes of strabismus range from the purely physical, such as lying on one side too much as a baby or a blow to the head, to the emotional. As you'll remember from Chapter 3, our right eye is associated with our analytical, dominant, masculine side, and the left eye with our creative, nurturing, female side. Considering your personality, your relationship with your parents, and the events that took place in your early life may throw light on how you developed this condition. You may find that Chapter 12, "Regression," will be helpful for you.

The case of Donna, a full-time mother who had been cross-eyed for all of her twenty-eight years, is a good illustration of the use of regression for strabismus. We didn't discover any emotional causes for her problem. However, she had a strong memory of lying in her crib on her stomach with her head turned to the right. She could feel her unsuccessful efforts to lift herself enough to turn her head. Through hypnotic suggestion I gave her infant-self this strength. For quite some time she imagined using the now-liberated right eye in that infantile situation. After the session her eyes were completely straight. It took another couple of months' work so that the right eye didn't turn if she was tired or stressed, but eventually the eye's ingrained habit became to remain straight.

Some optometrists use visual therapy techniques with children who suffer from strabismus, but surgery is often recommended. If you are considering this option for yourself or your child, be aware that it is usually unsuccessful. Even if the eyes do straighten out, it is usually only a cosmetic correction. The ability to fuse the two images into one coherent one is rarely regained. This may be due either to emotional reasons or to the simple fact that the surgery so damages the eye muscles that they can't regain their natural fusion ability. Even with the HypnoVision approach, I have had less success in helping people who have undergone surgery that with those who haven't.

Part of the problem with the surgery is the fact that the wrong muscle is attended to. The longer one is cut, a portion of it is removed, and then it is sewn back together. This muscle is not the problem, however. The *shorter* muscle is chronically tense. As soon as this muscle is relaxed, the eye straightens out properly. Most people with strabismus are aware of this, as they know the eye always turns more when they are tired or under stress.

Conversely, there is always an immediate straightening of the eye when vision improvement relaxation techniques are used. When possible, I enjoy giving five-day workshops. Invariably there is a person with strabismus in the group, and within the first few days the eye straightens out. However, before I added hypnosis to the program, the eye went right back into its old tension pattern as soon as the person was out of the environment of concentrated relaxation. Now the permanency of the change is increased because the subconscious remembers how to keep the eye straight and the fusion process intact.

If you also have myopia or hyperopia, you will follow the program already laid out for that problem with some modifications that will insure that your eyes become straight and fuse those two images into one. If strabismus is your only visual problem, you will still have an eight-week program so that your eyes have as much opportunity as possible to practice working as an aligned and coordinated team. I will lay out changes to be made in the myopia program. If you are hyperopic, add what follows here to the other changes laid out in the hyperopia program. If you have no problem with the clarity of your vision, omit all suggestions that refer to vision clarity as you add in the ones from this section.

WEEK ONE

In addition to the suggestions for week one of the myopic program (see pages 57–62), you will include specific ones for your strabismus. Whenever you see suggestions for the relaxation of your ciliary and oblique muscles, include your recti muscles as well. When you see suggestions for the shape of your eyes, add a suggestion that reads "Your recti muscles relax into equal lengths, and your eyes are straight and aligned." After the suggestion that you deserve clear vision, include another that states "You deserve perfectly aligned eyes and binocular vision." Affirm everywhere you can fit it in that "Your recti muscles are relaxed and aligned, and your eyes are straight." In the minisession (page 63) include your recti muscles in with the others that are mentioned. Also, add one suggestion that reads "I deserve perfect relaxed and aligned vision."

WEEK TWO

Simply use the massages and suggestions as they are given in the massage sessions for week two of the myopia program (see pages 64–75). The suggestions are general so there's no need to add any more specific ones. During the first of the two massages, you may very well discover that the muscles on the side of your body where your eye turns are tighter than on the other side. This is to be expected, so just give a little more attention to those tight muscles and you'll experience the extra needed relaxation in them and the corresponding eye.

WEEK THREE

During all three parts of the session for week three of the myopia program (see pages 75–85) you'll be adding some additional suggestions. During the first section, long swings, you will be performing two sets of these swings. The first time you go through them, you'll wear your eye patch on your good eye. If both eyes turn you won't need the patch unless one recovers more quickly than the other. Then do them once more, this time with both eyes uncovered. All eyes respond beautifully to the long swings, sunning, and short swings in this session, but yours will respond especially well to this relaxing series of moves. Make every effort to do the sunning swings in real sunlight. Its soothing powers are marvelous for straightening out eyes.

Everyplace you can work them in, add suggestions for the relaxation, balance, alignment, and straightening of your eyes. For the minisessions (page 84) add a suggestion that reads "My recti muscles are relaxed, balanced, and aligned, and my eyes work together as a coordinated team."

WEEK FOUR

This week you'll do the first of the visualization sessions exactly as written for the myopia program (see pages 86–89). These scenes are so relaxing that you'll find your eyes wonderfully straight afterward. For the minisession, add the same sentence that you did last week.

The second session is made up of healing visualizations (see pages 91–93) that you will change so that your recti will come into equal lengths. In this session make the same changes that you have been all along. In addition, insert the following suggestions during the healing massage visualization: "Visualize your four recti muscles connected to the eye that has been turning. Two of them are short and tense, pulling your eye out of alignment. See and feel the tightness. Now imagine the healing hands beginning to massage these tight recti muscles. They respond immediately to this deep, healing massage. . . . See and feel them softening, relaxing, stretching, and evening out in length. . . . It feels so good as these muscles let go, stretch and even out in their relaxation. . . . Softening, loosening, relaxing, stretching, evening. . . . As the muscles relax and stretch out to equal lengths, you can see and feel the pleasant straightening effect this has on your eye. More relaxed and straight than ever before. Your eyes can now work as an aligned, coordinated team."

WEEK FIVE

This week you will do your morning session from the myopia program (see pages 93–99) with your patch on your stronger eye, and then in the later session you will use both eyes. The suggestions will be the same for both sessions. However, if your day was so full of tension that your eye again turns radically, then again do the second session with the straight eye patched. Even though it is covered, the straighter eye will also benefit from the session. Also, when you are edging objects, do so only in the opposite direction of the turning of your eyes. For example, if your left eye turns in to the right corner of your eye, edge objects to your left so the eye will pull out toward the center. Add all the suggestions as before, and let your minisessions include one that reads "My recti muscles are relaxed, and my eyes are aligned." Also, on line 5 include "recti" with the reference to your oblique and ciliary muscles.

WEEK SIX

Week six of the myopia program will be the most challenging one for your strabismus, so we'll save it for next week. By then your eye that turns will have had more practice straightening out. This week you will do week seven of the myopia program (see pages 107–115). The only change you'll make is to go through the process twice, first with your good eye patched and then with both eyes together.

There's one important point to remember while working with the patch on your straighter eye. As you did with edging, you want to make sure that you turn your head enough to straighten out the eye as you are using it. Check your eyes in a mirror before you begin the exercise and see just how much you need to turn your head to make the eye straighter. Even if your eye has already straightened out by now, you still want to give it this extra practice working alone before you practice with both eyes. Don't forget to add the suggestions for your recti muscles and aligned eyes into the minisessions (see page 115).

If your session time coincides with a period when your eye has tired and pulled back out of alignment, you can add suggestions for it to relax and straighten out. Insert the same ones you have been using all along.

WEEK SEVEN

Now it's time to go back to week six of the myopia program (see pages 99–107) and achieve perfect fusion with your eyes. Do the session exactly as written but add the usual suggestions for your recti muscles relaxing and your eyes straightening. Add these suggestions often during the visualization and the exercise itself. By now your eyes and visual system should be up to the task of working together as a coordinated team. If, however, you discover that you can't achieve the optical illusions that accompany the fusion exercise, do only the visualization portion for a few days. When the mental part of your seeing is flawless, the physical part will follow suit. And, of course, make the usual additions to the minisessions (page 107).

WEEK EIGHT

As in the myopia program, this is a review week (see pages 116–127) so your eyes and visual system will fully integrate everything you've worked on so far. In both the full and the minisessions once again add the specific directions for the relaxation of your recti muscles and the alignment of your eyes every time there are references to your oblique and ciliary muscles.

Hopefully, you will have progressed to the point where you've made all the changes in your vision that you desired. However, as I mentioned earlier, this combination of problems sometimes takes longer to reverse than others. So stick with it, and use your pendulum to discover where you need to do more work.

Amblyopia

If one of your eyes has shut down to the point where it is considered legally blind, you'll follow the myopia program (see Chapter 6). Except for the work with string fusion you will do each exercise twice, once with the stronger eye patched and then again with both eyes. If time is a problem, you can spend just a short amount of time working both eyes together. If your good eye is so good that it doesn't need the myopia program, you'll do everything except the string fusion exercise with just the weaker eye, covering the good one with an eye patch. The sixth week develops fusion, which, of course, requires both eyes. If by week six you find the weak eye not yet strong enough to participate in this team effort, switch to week seven first so the eye will have more time to develop.

There is an additional suggestion that you will add to all your sessions. Whenever you come to references to the muscles of your eyes and the functioning of the optic center of your brain, you will add the following two sentences, filling in the blanks with "right" or "left" (the eye that turns): "The retina of your _____ eye is alive with energy, clearly records the images that come to it, and transmits these images to the optic center of your brain. The optic center of your brain interprets these images clearly and directs the retina of your _____ eye to function as fully as the your other one."

Cataracts

If your cataracts have not yet "ripened" to the point where you are a candidate for surgery, you may find you can reverse them through HypnoVision. Stay in close contact with your eye doctor so he or she can help you gauge your progress. During the five weeks that will make up your program, you may very well quite literally "see" significant improvement.

My favorite cataract client was Ellen, the epitome of the sweet great-grandmother. Ellen was terrified of surgery but had cataracts in both eyes that had progressed to the point where she could no longer drive and had to read with a magnifying glass. My initial reaction was simply to use hypnosis so that she would have a good surgical experience. But she was adamant about her aversion to any outside intervention. So we not only worked our way through the program as it is laid out here, but she was also wonderful about changing her life in every way that could affect her vision. She changed her diet, took vitamin supplements, practiced all the sessions at home, and even took up yoga. Against my advice she even did a headstand. She had to prop her feet against a wall, but she did her headstand every day. In three months she was again driving and reading with only the aid of her glasses. Ellen is my role model. If I can age as she has, my "golden years" will be just that.

WEEK ONE

Your first week will consist of the same one for the presbyopia program (see pages 132–136) with a few added suggestions. Whenever you see suggestions for the moisture, circulation, and flexibility of your lenses, insert the word "clear" before "lenses."

WEEK TWO

This week is also essentially the same as week two of the presbyopia program (see pages 136–147). Again, expand the suggestions for your lenses so that they include the word "clear."

WEEK THREE

This week you switch over to the myopia program and use its week three (see pages 75–85). The swings in this session are wonderfully stimulating for the circulation in your lenses. If you saw clearly in the distance before you developed cataracts, you can remove the suggestions for relaxing the oblique and ciliary muscles and seeing clearly in the distance. Substitute instead a suggestion that reads "Your lenses are clear, moist, and flexible, and you see clearly at all distances."

The sunning swings are wonderful for healing cataracts. However, if you find yourself too sensitive to sunlight to do them outside, use an indoor light.

During the short swing segment of this exercise, there is a visualization for seeing a three-by-five card in the distance. If your distance vision needs work too, use the visualization the way it is. If not, imagine that you are seeing a one-by-two card only a foot in front of you. If you wear bifocals or trifocals, switch back and forth from the distance card to the near card.

WEEK FOUR

Staying with the myopia program now, you'll do the same first session as for week four (see pages 85–90). The beautiful nature scenes in this session are beneficial to all vision problems. As you relax and imagine what is described, the healing circulation will open even more into your lenses. If you would like to stimulate your near vision as well as your distance vision, imagine that you occasionally pick up a magazine and see it clearly. Beforehand choose a page of a magazine with a picture and a little print on it that you will be able to remember.

You will be adding some extra emphasis to the healing of your lenses when you do the second full session (pages 91–93). When you visualize the massage portion of this section, take out the references to oblique and ciliary muscles, unless you are also nearsighted, and concentrate on the massage of your lenses. See them beginning as cloudy and becoming clear. To the minisession script supplied in the myopia program, add this suggestion: "My lenses are clear, moist, and flexible."

WEEK FIVE

Eyes with cataracts tense up and lose the natural movement that clear vision requires. This week is the same for week five of the myopia program (see pages 93–99), and will return that movement to your visual system. Whenever you see a reference to your lenses, expand it to include "clear." If you want to stimulate your near vision as well as your distance vision, use a magazine or calendar picture for part of the exercise. Add suggestions for your clear, flexible lenses shifting into a concave shape for nearpoint vision.

If you have not achieved a significant clearing of your cataracts by the fifth week, use your pendulum. Modify the questions at the end of the myopia chapter (page 127) by asking your subconscious for answers to 1, 2 (if yes, then 2a, 2e, 2f, 2g, 2h), 3, 4, and 5. In addition, if you received a "yes" answer for 2, ask yourself also: Do I need to improve my diet? Do I need more physical exercise?

Glaucoma

While you may find that HypnoVision works miracles for your glaucoma, let me emphasize how important it is to continue the medical supervision of this condition. Glaucoma can sneak up on you and do considerable damage before it actually shows up in your vision. Don't take chances with a condition that can easily lead to blindness. However, even if HypnoVision doesn't turn out to be the answer for you, the program poses no risk to your condition provided you still follow doctor's orders.

Like cataracts, glaucoma responds to techniques that promote relaxation, circulation, and movement into the eyes. You will, in fact, use the same format as the previous section on cataracts. What will change is the specific suggestions and visualizations. You don't need anything directed to either myopia or cataracts in terms of the muscles and the lenses. You will be making suggestions for the canal of Schlemm to open and close freely and regularly so that the aqueous humor enters and leaves the anterior chamber of your eye every four hours as it is supposed to. When you visualize your eyes receiving a healing massage, you will picture the canals of Schlemm being restored to optimal health and functioning by the healing hands. When you visualize the golden healing energy, let it be like a laser beam that cleans and opens the canal. Remember that the canal is a tube in the lining of the eye, so see that light encircling your eyeball.

Macular Degeneration

If you are suffering from macular degeneration, the whole thrust of your HypnoVision program will be to reactivate the cones in the center of your retinas, the maculae, and to convince the optic center of your brain to keep this area working. Even if aging is behind the degeneration, you can arrest and possibly reverse the condition. You will follow the five-step program given above for cataracts, only with your own special additions.

Take out all references to the mechanics of myopia and cataracts, and replace them with suggestions for the regeneration of your cones and the clarity of your central, detailed vision. During the massage session in the week two, when you massage your shoulders add a suggestion that this stimulates your retinas. Everywhere you can fit it in, suggest that healing energy is returning life and function to the nerve cells in your maculae, that your central vision is regenerating, and that the optic center of your brain constantly stimulates your retinas, especially the maculae, to function optimally. When you are visualizing healing hands giving a massage, keep the massage on your retinas. When you are visualizing golden healing energy, see it stimulating your retinas. You'll be pleased with how your mind can restore your vision.

I've witnessed remarkable visual recoveries of macular degeneration through HypnoVision. But if you don't respond as much as you'd like in the first five weeks, use your pendulum, with the questions for cataracts as a guideline, and see what extra work you should do.

Retinitis Pigmentosa

If you're suffering from retinitis pigmentosa, the object of your HypnoVision program will be to restore life and energy to the cones and, especially, the rods on the outer areas of your retinas. However, as with glaucoma, it is important to continue medical supervision for this condition. So even if HypnoVision doesn't turn out to be the answer for you, it poses no risk to your condition, provided you still follow doctor's orders. The same process of relaxation, circulation, movement, and visualization as you will find in the previous section on cataracts applies to you. However, you won't give suggestions for the mechanics of either myopia or cataracts, you'll supply ones that will reactivate the full functioning of your retinas.

Replace every suggestion that doesn't apply to your condition with ones that will stimulate your retinas. State that they are vibrantly alive, completely energized, and function optimally. Affirm that your brain sends messages to your retinas for all the rods and cones to activate and record light and images. Be sure to include these suggestions in the minisessions too. When you visualize healing massage and energy, suggest and see this concentrated around the outer edges of your retinas.

If your eyes don't respond in five weeks, it is most likely that you simply need to repeat the program. Check with your pendulum to see if any specific part of the program will be especially helpful, using the questions for cataracts as a guideline.

11

Working with a Partner

Working with a partner can lead to the greatest successes. You can, of course, simply tape the sessions and then follow them with someone, but the presence of a live hypnotist so increases the effectiveness of the suggestions that it is worth the extra time to trade back and forth in the roles. Not only will each of you benefit from having a personal hypnotist, but to some degree hypnotists always "get" the positive suggestions they give to others. So, in effect, you can get more work done in the same amount of time. This doesn't necessarily mean that you will finish in less time, but it does mean that you may accomplish deeper changes during the program than if you were going it alone.

The foremost requirement for the success of a partner experience is that you stick to business. The camaraderie of a friendship can be a great morale booster, but you don't want to work with a friend if it will distract you from the work to be done. In the HypnoVision program, you will not be just teammates. You will be alternating roles of hypnotist and subject, so your roles will be very like that of teacher and student. When I was a high school English teacher, I learned quickly that being friends with my students had to be an extracurricular activity. Otherwise the classroom, educational situation deteriorated into friendly but unproductive chit-chat. And I have since witnessed this same phenomenon numerous times when I helped set up partner homework among my clients. Those who don't firmly establish that the sessions are for working have a fun time but don't improve their vision much at all. Don't fall into this seductive trap!

To work with a partner, it's not necessary that you have similar vision, but it can be helpful. This way the suggestions you give to each other truly have a chance to sink in during both of your roles. On the other hand, don't worry that giving somebody else suggestions that are very different from those you need will have an adverse effect on you. Your subconscious isn't that naive. Also, your conscious awareness that the suggestions aren't meant for you will filter out anything that doesn't apply.

Anyone can hypnotize anyone else provided you are both willing participants in this joint effort. Remember that it's not a competition. The hypnotist does not "do something" to the subject. The person in the role of the hypnotist is the guide, but the success of the journey depends primarily on the willing cooperation of the subject. The old axiom that all hypnosis is self-hypnosis is definitely true. Everything that goes on happens within the subject's mind. It's just easier if you have someone helping along the way. Having said that, let me emphasize that the more skilled you become as a hypnotist, the more you can help your partner succeed. There are two primary qualities you want to develop, a good speaking voice and a confident tone in that voice. You want to speak slowly, clearly, and rhythmically and keep your voice within the lower parts of its range. And you want to sound as if you have absolute confidence in what you are saying. You are the trusted authority figure, so sound like it. Not artificially, though. You're not trying to sound like anybody else, just the you that is comfortable and reassuring to be around.

Practice, of course, makes perfect or, at least, improved. While it is certainly okay if you choose to work only with the scripts for the actual programs, you may find the practice exercises in this chapter very helpful in developing your confidence in your role as the hypnotist. Additionally, playing with these exercises will also increase your skill as a subject. Have fun with them, for they are opportunities to develop the focused concentration and creative imagination that it takes to excel as a subject. It bears repeating that the hypnotist does not do anything to the subject other than guide the experience. The experience happens inside the subject. Let it happen inside you, let your imagination create a new reality, and you'll be able to access the depths of your subconscious mind where real changes can take place. When you are the hypnotist, be there as a steady guiding force. After you practice these skills, I'll detail paired exercises that you can add to the HypnoVision programs presented in earlier chapters to make them even more effective.

The first practice session, to be done over and over until you both feel comfortable and accomplished at it, is the one in Chapter 5 on pages 46–50. The leisurely pace of the induction and deepening will give you time to develop each of your roles as hypnotist and subject. When you feel ready, use the following short session to reinforce your skills. It involves physical contact and visible responses to the suggestions, which demonstrates to both hypnotist and subject that the hypnotic state is being entered. If you become so good at them as a subject that you enter what feels like a deep state of hypnosis, use them in actual sessions to shorten the induction and deepening time. You may find, in fact, that you go much deeper with this technique than with either the long induction or the rapid one. In most cases, whenever a hypnotist has physical contact with a subject the trance state is deep and immediate. This is partly why stage hypnotists seem to have such an effect on their subjects.

After the induction the hypnotist will guide the subject through a series of three suggestions. First, however, it is best to practice just the induction three or four times before adding the suggestion sections. There is too, of course, an awakening procedure to go through.

For the induction the subject will sit comfortably and keep his or her head level. The hypnotist holds one hand flat and parallel to the subject's face, about two inches out from and three inches above the subject's head. The tip of the little finger is in line with the center of the subject's forehead. As the subject you will feel quite a significant straining pull on your eyes as you look up at the hypnotist's hand.

Now let your creative imagination take over as you follow these instructions from the hypnotist:

o

"Focus your eyes on the tip of my little finger. Keep focused on it, and don't even blink unless you really have to. Notice that your eyes don't like looking up at this angle. Notice that your eyes are becoming tired. Tired and heavy. Very tired and very heavy. So heavy. You can barely keep your eyes open. So heavy, you can barely keep your eyes open. In a moment I'm going to pass my hand down in front of your face. Keep your eyes focused on the tip of my little finger. As I pass my hand down in front of your face, the tired, heavy weight of your eyelids will pull your eyes closed [slowly move your hand downward, just in front of your subject's face, keeping the movement going until you see the eyes close]. . . . Eyes so heavy and tired. Let the weight of your lids pull them closed. When they close you relax deeply. So heavy and tired and lazy. Eyes closed, completely relaxed. So relaxed [the subject's neck will now most likely relax so that the head is hanging forward]. . . . Let your eyelids feel even heavier now. Heavy, loose, and limp. So heavy that no matter how hard you try to open your eyes, they just won't budge. Try to open your eyes and notice that they are too heavy and limp to open. Give up the effort and feel yourself sink into even deeper relax-ation. . . . Wonderfully relaxed. . . . In a moment I'll count from one to three. Each number will signal your conscious mind to return to full wakening consciousness. When I count the number three you'll be fully alert, feeling relaxed and refreshed. . . . One—coming up. Two—more alert, deepen your breaths. . . . Three—all the way up. Wide awake and alert when you open your eyes. Feeling refreshed. . . ."

o

After you've gone over this enough to where you both feel comfort-able with your roles, use the following script after you have com-pleted the hand passing and heavy eyelid process:

o

"... Extend your arms straight out in front of you now, palms facing each other about a foot apart. ... In a moment I'm going to place powerful magnets in the palms of your hands. These magnets will pull your hands together. When I place them in your palms, feel the magnetic pull [press your thumbs into the centers of the subject's palms, then remove your hands]. ... Feel the magnets pulling your hands together. Your hands moving and closing. Your hands moving and closing as the magnets pull them together [keep repeating "moving and closing" if the hands aren't moving steadily toward one another]. ... When your hands touch and you sink even deeper into hypnotic relaxation, let them relax down into your lap [give the subject time for the hands to come together; when they do the subject will visibly relax even more]. ... Good. ... Now imagine that your right hand is becoming light. So light that it is beginning to float up. So light that it feels like there is a helium balloon tied to the wrist of your right hand. Your arm will bend at the wrist as the balloon lifts it up. ... What would it feel like if your right hand was floating up? Lighter and lighter. Floating up. Your wrist being lifted by a helium balloon. Your hand and arm limp. Lighter and lighter. Floating up. Up and up [allow time for the gradual lifting of the arm, repeating "lighter and lighter" if necessary]. ... Your arm remains suspended, floating, and light. ... Now the balloon is released from your wrist. Bring your hand down to your lap now, and relax more deeply when it touches your leg. ... So wonderfully relaxed. ... I'll count from one to three now. Each number up will bring you back to full waking consciousness. When I count the last number you'll be wide awake, wonderfully rested and refreshed. One—coming up. Two—almost alert. Three—eyes open, take in a deep breath, wide awake and alert, feeling rested and refreshed."

o

For most of the program you will simply use the scripts that have already been supplied. They are full of carefully chosen words and phrases, but you still have the option of adapting them to your own speaking pattern. Additionally, as you go along you may discover other suggestions that have individual importance to you. Do be creative and tailor the basic programs to your own needs. However, be absolutely certain that you phrase your suggestions so they are positive rather than negative. For reasons not fully understood, the subconscious tends to omit negatives. For example, if you say "You are not as myopic as before," your subconscious will hear "You are myopic." Phrased correctly, the suggestion should read something like "Your sight is clearer than before."

If you use Chapter 12, "Regression," you have a chance as the hypnotist to go far beyond the script given. By listening carefully to the subject talk about the past, you may be able to come up with additional questions that can be helpful in both uncovering and letting go of these past incidents. But be very careful that you don't interject your own opinions and beliefs. You are a caring questioner, not the judge of how the subject should think and feel. If you find it appropriate to make up suggestions as you work through memories with the subject, again, make sure they are phrased positively. Let's say, for example, that you want to reinforce lack of fearfulness of seeing clearly. You wouldn't say "You're not afraid to see clearly," you'd say instead "You have the confidence to see clearly."

Perhaps the most interesting, and potentially beneficial, activities you can do as a team are massages. Several massages that require two people were omitted from the programs. I use them all the time in my practice, and they are enjoyable and effective. I will lay them out here for you in the same series I use, but if you want to separate them and use them with other parts of the program, that's fine too. Used in the way I'll describe, they make up a whole session, one that you can repeat periodically throughout the program when you have extra time. An ideal situation would be to use them right after the standard shoulder, neck, and face massage. It will serve as a warmup for what you will find to be a very powerful session. They are also excellent to use after the induction in any session, before continuing with the rest of the suggestions. Whenever you use them, make sure the subject is hypnotized so they will have maximum effectiveness.

You'll want to memorize this script as it's very difficult to massage and read at the same time. After you have directed the subject through the self-massage or the induction before another session, leave out the palming suggestions and go on in this manner:

o

"Keeping your eyes closed, lie down now, and feel yourself relax even more. In a moment I'm going to massage your forehead. As I do you will relax deeply, and this massage will further release all tension from your eyes and visual system. The instant I touch my fingers to your forehead, you will relax more deeply [place the first three fingers of your hand just above the bridge of the subject's nose, slightly above the eyebrow line on what is known as the "third eye"]. . . . More deeply relaxed. . . . As I massage you will feel relaxation and healing energy flowing into your eyes and visual system. [With your wrist loose and your fingertips still gently touching the subject's skin, begin a constant shaking, vibratory movement. Hold your fingers in one place and shake from the wrist. Keep this up throughout.] Constant, vibrating waves of relaxation and energy flowing into your eyes and visual system. . . . More visual relaxation than you've ever experienced. . . . Deeper and deeper into hypnotic, healing relaxation. . . . Your visual system is relaxed, energized, and healed [here you can insert specifics, such as the oblique muscles letting go, the eyes returning to the shape for clear vision, the lenses flooded with healing circulation, etc.]. . . . This massage is healing your vision. . . . Clear sight restored. . . . Feel the massage loosening your eye muscles. . . . Feel healing energy flowing throughout your visual system. . . . Feel the vibration of energy in your eyes. Feel it flow down your optic nerves and into the optic center of your brain. . . . Everything in your eyes and visual system is balanced and healed by this energy. . . . Your sight is energized, relaxed, and clear [go over and over these suggestions for about five minutes].... In a moment I'll remove my fingers from your forehead and you'll feel the healing power of the massage spreading even more deeply through your entire visual system [slow the vibrating movement to a standstill, then let your fingers rest a moment on the subject's forehead before you remove them].... Feel the healing energy in your visual system.... Your visual system is now ready to release all blocks to perfect vision.... Keeping your eyes closed, come into a seated position with your head relaxed forward. [You may want to gently assist the subject in sitting up. When the subject is seated with head relaxed in a forward and down position, kneel to one side so that you can have room to stretch the palms of your hands out over the base of the subject's spine. Don't actually make physical contact, but hold your hands next to each other about two inches from the subject's spine. Begin a continual series of hand passes up

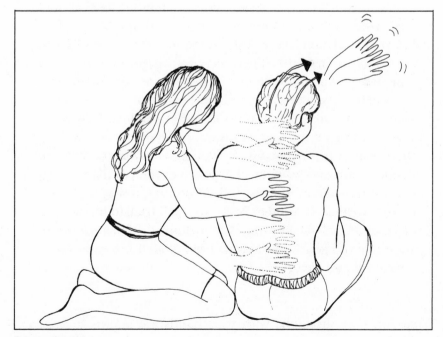

Energy Sweep

the spine and over the head, always passing from top to bottom and bringing your hands all the way over the head rather than up in the air directly above the spine. You are sweeping energy up the spine, through any blocks. Each time you finish a pass, flick your hands into the air—this will relax your hands and throw off any of the energy blocks that have emerged. You will do this for about five minutes. Let your exhalations coincide with the hand passes].... Energy flowing.... Blocks being swept away.... Feel the energy moving through you, sweeping through the blocks.... Energy released and flowing.... Feel the energy flowing up your spine, into the optic center of your brain, into your optic nerves, into your eyes, and through your closed lids.... A free flow of healing energy.... Visual system opening and clearing and healing.... Your vision is energized, relaxed, and clear [give the specifics again that apply to the program you are working with].... Energy flows freely up your spine, into the optic center of your brain, down your optic nerves, and into your eyes.... Your vision is balanced, healed, and energized.... Your vision is energized, relaxed, and clear [go over and over these suggestions while you make hand passes for five minutes. Then relax your hands down].... In a moment I'll count from one to five. With each number up you will become more alert and more aware of the freedom in your visual system. On the number five you'll be fully alert, vision clear, feeling wonderfully energized.... One—feeling the energy within your visual system. Two—as you breathe deeper your energy rises. Three—feel the circulation and energy in your eyes. Four—sight so free, energized, and clear. On the next number bring yourself back to full waking alertness. Five—all the way back. Blink softly as you open your eyes and gently swing your head from side to side. Sight energized and clear."

o

What you have just done with your hands are known as *mesmeric passes.* They are very like some of those used by Franz Mesmer. We don't yet fully understand the energy fields in and around our bodies, but we do know that they exist and are powerful. As mentioned earlier, Dr. Esdaile used mesmeric passes over wounded patients in India and achieved both anesthesia and improved healing without any suggestions. In my own experience I have seen remarkable changes in vision after these passes are made. In fact, they were responsible for my first experience with a dramatic moment of visual healing. It was during the first Bates workshop I attended. We had worked in groups of three, two of us at a time doing passes over the third person. We could all feel the hands passing over us even though we were never touched, but one woman had a much more significant experience. When she opened her eyes we were all startled to hear shouts of "I can see! I can see!" It sounded like something out of a faith-healing revival meeting. Her vision remained crystal clear for the remainder of the day.

Ever since I incorporated hypnosis into the mesmeric passes, I've seen these spontaneous bursts of clear vision afterward more and more. In addition to using the procedure along with the other massage, this combination of vibration and hand passes is extremely beneficial at the end of the program. When sight has already improved to a great extent, this session can sweep away the last vestiges of the problem and culminate in a more complete recovery.

One more technique that you can do as partners can have a profound impact on your vision. You can stage one or more marathon sessions. These can last anywhere from four to eight hours depending on your stamina and ability to maintain your concentration. You can use all or parts of the whole program that you are working on. The subject will remain hypnotized the entire time, even when having a snack or taking a bathroom break. By the way, the hypnotist should schedule such breaks every now and then so that the subject doesn't have any conscious thought of needs occurring.

You're not expected to be the hypnotist the whole time. Even I don't do that in marathon workshops that I lead. You can take rest breaks by playing tapes of some of the sessions that you have recorded ahead of time. You can also bring in someone else as an additional hypnotist. And you can keep the mood of concentrated relaxation going with the aid of soft background music. The right music can greatly enhance healing. The genre known as "New Age" includes many selections that are perfect for healing hypnosis. I use this music during most of my sessions, whether they are marathons or one hour. For workshops I am fortunate enough to have live background music that complements every nuance of my voice and suggestions provided by an enormously talented musician. He also happens to be my husband, so I am doubly blessed.

Not many of the clients that I've paired up have managed to organize marathons for themselves, but those that have taken place produced dramatic results. For example, Lisa and Mary, both myopes, were each able to pass the vision test for their driver's licenses after a full day's marathon. Their birthdays were only days apart, so they chose the occasion to see what they could accomplish. That one day produced the 20 percent improvement they each needed to see 20/40.

For me, marathons with individuals are rare because of the scheduling and cost involved. But I often see as much improvement in two- or five-day workshops as I would expect to occur in a month or more of private work. The dramatic effects don't always last, but progress becomes much quicker. If you can find the time, it will be well worth the effort.

One of the best advantages of working with a partner is sharing the celebration of your success. Nobody else will understand so well what you have accomplished. Do something special!

12

Regression

If your subconscious and your pendulum have determined that remembering your past will be beneficial to your vision, regression will be an important and potentially transforming experience for you. Your present maturity and the hypnotic trance will combine forces so that this will be an exercise in remembering rather than an act of reliving. You may feel emotions and even be moved to tears, but you will feel distanced from the experience, as if you were watching a movie. The truth is that you survived whatever occurred earlier, and it is from this vantage point of the mature survivor that you will view your past. In addition, if there really is something that would be too difficult to deal with at this point, your subconscious will simply shield you by keeping the memory hidden for now. Forget all that nonsense you have seen in movies and on television!

For the vast majority of you, the formative events that will surface in your memory will not be all that traumatic. The most common events I uncover with clients are family arguments and frictions, overly strict religious upbringing, and shyness in school. It was not so much *what* happened as it was our reaction to what happened. Most myopes, for example, didn't suffer through events any different from most clearsighted people. We just habitually responded to stressful situations by fearfully pulling inward, both emotionally and visually. The regression exercise will, no doubt, be very interesting to you and quite possibly emotional, but the skill you will gain from the session is even more important. By remembering how you reacted at the visual level, you'll be able to change that ingrained response pattern. As you perceive the events in a new light, your perspective will quite literally change.

But, of course, not everyone has mere anxieties behind his or her visual malfunction. I've worked with a wide range of truly traumatic causative factors, such as alcoholic or otherwise dysfunctional families, sexual abuse, and child abuse. Hypnosis is the ideal means of coming to grips with and then shedding the legacy of these deeper problems. However, this is not something I recommend you to do on your own, or even with a partner. This is when you need a qualified and well-recommended hypnotherapist. I'm not discounting other forms of therapy should you desire them, but I am, of course, biased toward my own field due to the miracles I've seen worked through it. But the point to remember is that this regression session is set up to restructure your visual response pattern, it is not meant as emotional therapy. If you feel you need that, get such help before you do this session so that your subconscious will be free to do the work of visual changing. And remember, this is an exercise of memory, not one of reliving.

It is not at all difficult to regress yourself, but as with all hypnotic experiences, it can be beneficial to work with a partner. Not only do we tend to relax more deeply if we let a trusted person guide us through the experience, but this person can also be very helpful if he or she listens attentively and has good instincts. A good, objective second party can often pick up on what questions should be asked and what additional suggestions would be helpful to the process of getting beyond and setting to rest the past.

Still, I know most of you will be doing this on your own, so the script I have created will enable you to travel back and heal your past as well as your visual response to it. In addition to the taped script, you may want to have another tape recorder handy. You will not go

so deeply into the hypnotic state that you will later be unaware of
what you remembered or said, but it is often useful to listen to your
responses later. Use a small, portable tape recorder and have it very
close to your head or even in one hand so you can bring it right to
your mouth when you speak. The first time I was regressed I was
later astounded that the rest of the group had not been able to hear
my interaction with the hypnotist. When we are hypnotized, we
think we are speaking more loudly than we actually are, so keep that
microphone very close by.

A variety of methods can be used to induce regression. I have
chosen one that involves a beautiful visualization so that you will
have an additional opportunity to develop this skill so vital to clear
sight. Even if you have become so proficient at quickly entering and
deepening your hypnotic state that you've been using the rapid
induction for the full sessions, using the complete induction here
will relax away any lingering qualms that might otherwise interfere
with the depth of your hypnotic state. After this induction, go on
with the following script. Palming is optional.

o

"Imagine that you are sitting on a magic carpet that is floating high in the sky. . . . See the colors and patterns on your
carpet. Touch it and feel its texture. . . . All around you is a
beautiful blue sky. One fleecy white cloud floats by you. . . .
You feel good about the time-traveling adventure you are
about to embark on. You are confident that you will have
clear, accurate memories and that you are completely emotionally competent to see your past for what it was and let go
of its grip on your vision. You are a mature, confident adult,
no longer that young, impressionable person of the past.
This is an exercise of your memory, not a reliving of past
events. . . . Imagine looking over the edge of your magic
carpet to the earth below you. The landscape you see is one
of rolling green hills, dotted with trees and flowers. A wide
river is running through a valley beneath you. In one direction this river leads to the future, and in the other it leads to the

past. . . . Your carpet is beginning to move now, following the river as it flows into the past. . . . The river flows back to the past and so do you. . . . Experience the sense of movement. . . . Farther and farther back. . . . Years are flying by as you move back into the past. . . . Flowing with the river back into your past. . . . In a few moments you'll be back to an event in your past when you shut down your vision as an emotional response to what was happening. I'll count down from three to one, and when you hear the number one you'll be at that event. You will remember it clearly, but you will remain detached, as if you were viewing this event on a movie screen. Three—moving back. Two—farther back. When you hear the next number you'll be there. One—remembering *now* a scene where you didn't want to see what was happening. But you did see it, and now you remember it clearly. . . . How old are you? [Respond to the questions out loud if you have a second tape recorder or a partner.] . . . Where are you? . . . What are you wearing? . . . Who else is there? . . . What is happening? . . . As you remember this event, you observe it from the vantage point of a mature, emotionally developed adult. . . . At the same time you can feel the eyes of that young person who was you visually contracting in some way, trying to shut out the view. Experience that visual response. Feel your shoulders, neck, jaws, and eyes tense up. . . . Feel the tension in the part of your eyes that developed your particular visual problem. [Insert here those particulars. For example, the oblique extraocular muscles of myopes tightening and squeezing the eyeballs out of the shape for clear vision.] . . . As you do, realize that there was nothing to be gained by this response. The event happened anyway, and you were emotionally affected by it anyway, so nothing was gained by shutting off part of your visual process. . . . With that awareness in mind, replay this scene. This time see and feel yourself responding so that there is no need to tense your visual system. . . . What could you say or do instead of restricting your vision? . . . You could even simply look the other way, for example, and rest your gaze on something you like seeing. You can also respond emotionally to the event while still seeing it clearly. Shutting off your vision didn't change what happened. What could you have done instead? . . . As you respond this way in your mind, the optic center of your brain directs your eyes to see clearly in this situation and all others. As you imagine responding differently than you did in the past, feel your shoulders, neck, jaws, and eyes relaxing. . . . This feels so much better. . . . This is the natural response of healthy clear sight. It feels so much better. . . . Allowing your vision to remain relaxed and clear in spite of the events taking place is once again your natural instinctive visual response. . . . Allowing your vision to remain relaxed and clear in spite of what is happening around you is once again your natural instinctive visual response. . . . This past event is behind you. You survived, and you've grown and matured. You are a worthwhile human being, and you deserve clear vision. You are no longer trapped and constricted, visually or emotionally, by this event in your past. . . . Feel the sense of freedom and expansion that this knowledge brings. . . . Relaxed clarity of vision is your natural, instinctive visual response. . . . It's okay to see clearly. . . . It's okay to see clearly. . . . Your vision is free, relaxed, and clear. . . . In a few moments I'll once again count down from three to one. When I count the number one, you'll be back to another event in your past to which you responded by restricting your vision. Three—going back. Two—almost there. You'll remember the event vividly when I count the next number. One— clearly remember another incident in which you responded by blocking out part of your vision. . . . How old are you? . . . Where are you? . . . Who else is there? . . . What is happening? . . . As you remember the experience, once again feel your visual response, the tightening of your shoulders, neck, jaws, and eyes, the restriction of your visual field. [Insert again the particulars that apply to you.] . . . Recognize once again that this response served no real purpose. The event still happened, you were still emotionally affected by it. Yet you survived and went on with your life. You not only survived but you have also grown and matured. The past is behind you. . . . Look at this incident with your renewed visual response. Feel your shoulders, neck, jaws, and eyes remaining relaxed [mention those specifics again, stressing their relaxation] . . . your vision clear. . . . This natural positive visual response pattern is again yours. . . . There's nothing to be gained by shutting down your vision. . . . Feel the sense of freedom and expansion, emotionally and visually. . . . Your past is just that, past. . . . You view your past as a learning experience. . . . You have learned, matured, grown. You have within you reserves of personal power that you've never fully recognized before. Experience how it feels to acknowledge your own personal power. . . . You are a powerful person who has prevailed over negative situations in your life. . . . You now acknowledge and accept your own personal power. Through doing so you now release your old negative visual response pattern. The blockages to clear vision have vanished. . . . You are free. Your vision is free. . . . Your vision is free and functions with relaxed spontaneity, and you see clearly. . . . It's okay to see clearly, and you are ready for clear vision. . . . The more clearly you see, the more you are able to handle any situation that arises. . . . It feels so good to be free to see clearly. . . . You see clearly, and it feels so very good. . . . In a few moments I'll begin counting from one to five. At the subconscious level each number up will reinforce the renewed freedom, power, and clarity of your vision. At the conscious level the numbers will serve as signals that it is time to return to fully alert consciousness, and by the number five you'll be wide awake, alert, and refreshed. One—a feeling of coming up, free and refreshed. Your breaths beginning to deepen as you draw energy in. Two—energy flowing, feeling your own personal power. Three—halfway up. Feel the freedom and moisture in your eyes. Four—almost all the way back. You have regenerated your personal power and you can feel it in your eyes. When I count the next number, bring yourself all the way back to full waking consciousness, alert and refreshed. Five—all the way back. Take in a deep breath and stretch. When you open your eyes, blinking softly and swinging your head gently from side to side, you'll be fully alert, filled with confidence, and your vision free and clear."

o

Some people need only one session to remember key events, reconcile them with their present maturity, and free up their visual system. Most of us, however, need to do a little more remembering and a little more mental practicing of being able to see these events without the visual constriction. Three times is about the average. You can check with your pendulum to see if your visual system and emotions have really made the adjustments.

Occasionally when I regress people to find out about the initial events that shaped their visual response pattern, another entire category of memories crops up. The first time it happened I was taken completely by surprise. The woman began crying out in pain and then exclaimed, "They're putting my eyes out!" She had spontaneously regressed to a past lifetime and had a vivid recollection of being blinded by hot pokers, apparently in punishment for witnessing a sacred ritual that nobody of her class was allowed to see. This was particularly interesting in light of the fact that this woman had still exhibited enormous tension around her eyes in spite of several months of work with me. After this experience her eyes relaxed immediately and she made rapid visual improvement. Since then I have been with a handful of people when they had memories of this sort, fortunately none as gruesome as the first one, and they all made the same rapid improvements after the experience.

This, of course, brings up the whole concept of reincarnation. If you believe in it, there is some chance that a prior life's event is reflected by the current condition of your sight. But it's strictly a matter of belief. If you are quite certain that you are here only this time around, you won't have past-life recollections. Personally, the concept of our potentials taking many lifetimes to grow and develop makes sense to me. Through my own regressions I have garnered valuable information about my current personality and life situations. But I obviously won't know if this is my creative imagination or the real thing until I pass out of this life. What I do know is that I have gained beneficial insights that have improved the quality of my life. And this is how I judge all other belief systems. If they are helpful without becoming obsessive in a person's life, then they are worthwhile and positive.

Regardless of your perspective, looking into and reconciling your past is an experience well worth the effort. That old adage about how we are doomed to repeat the past if we do not learn from its lessons is a truism if ever there was one. So be brave, you have nothing to lose but your negative habit patterns, visual and emotional.

13

HypnoSports:
Vision Games for All Eyes

HypnoSports aren't an official requirement for your program, but you'll help your spirits and your sight if you indulge in some visual fun as often as possible. Playing or watching games that keep your eyes moving, especially games involving balls, can be a wonderful help to your sight. On the other hand, if your eyes fall right back into their old patterns of tensing in order to see, there will be little or no benefit. I've always included ball-tossing games in my workshops and encouraged my private clients to engage in some games on their own. But not until I learned the importance of subconscious suggestion did I realize that it was needed in order to break the negative habits of vision in both games and everyday life.

HypnoSports are any for which you can hypnotize yourself beforehand in order to play the game (in your waking state, of course!) focused on your vision as opposed to winning. The more noncompetitive, the better. A leisurely pace will also encourage your eyes to use their new skills rather than to revert back to the old tense ones. My newest invention and current favorite at this point is HypnoBadminton (I'll just stick Hypno on anything, won't I!).

227

Badminton is slow and sets are inexpensive. In fact, the cheaper the better, since these come supplied with plastic birdies in bright colors that are easy to see. As I wrote this book I often emerged from my office only twice a day: once for a walk and once for a rousing game of slow-motion badminton. Before each game I briefly hypnotized myself and reminded my tired eyes that now was their chance to loosen up their focus while I relaxed my mind and moved around a bit. I also reminded my extraocular and ciliary muscles when to relax and when to contract. To make the game even more relaxing, my husband and I kept score by making the first person to reach twenty-one the *loser.* The object of the game was to keep the birdie in play rather than hit shots that couldn't be returned. And most important, I remembered to keep my eyes on the birdie, following its path from the surface of my racket all the way to my husband's and back again.

You can apply this idea to any game. Ping-Pong and tennis are also good choices, but not if they are too fast for you or if you can't yet see the ball without glasses. Ball tossing, Frisbee throwing, paddle tennis, racquetball, and even watching sports on TV are also possibilities.

If you are nearsighted you want to look for activities where you are on your feet and moving. Myopes tend to have what I call poor eye-foot coordination. We are more in our heads than in our bodies, and the result is a lack of being "grounded." Psychically and physically we don't have our feet on the ground. It takes a bit of effort at first, but if you remember both to follow the ball with your eyes and let your feet lead you to where it is coming, you'll find that you improve both your vision and your skill at the game. The more you hypnotize yourself beforehand and affirm this coordination, the easier it will come.

No matter what kind of vision you have, your pregame suggestions should also include a reminder to breathe and blink as you play. In the past you tensed up these reflexes when you made an effort to see. Now the breathing and blinking will help your eyes relax and function optimally.

Keeping your eyes on the constantly moving object is of paramount importance. Not only will this improve your playing (ask any athlete), but it will also dramatically help your vision. With just this one object to focus on, your visual system will respond by functioning with spontaneous efficiency. Your eyes will loosen up and naturally begin to shift their focus in and out properly. Give yourself suggestions for keeping your eyes on the ball (or birdie) at all times, and repeat them to yourself while you are playing.

If possible, verbalize the suggestions out loud as you play. If you're myopic, for example, you can say "Eyes and lenses rounding as I follow the ball into the distance." If you're hyperopic, you can remind yourself "Eyes and lenses narrowing as I watch the ball come to me." Presbyopes would affirm "Lenses shifting shape as I watch the ball come in and go out." Any way you choose to word suggestions so they work for you is fine. Even single words that you associate with what your eyes need to do are good reinforcement, such as "round" or "longer." I sometimes sound as if I'm chanting a mantra as I give a good posthypnotic workout to my eyes. "Posthypnotic" is an important point. It was one thing to stand for some lazy long swings while hypnotized, but you want to be fully alert when you play HypnoSports. Be sure to count yourself up into full alertness before you begin. And remember the spirit of play! I'm confident that you'll experience improvements in your vision each time you play a HypnoSport!

If you would like information on Lisette Scholl's workshops or on tapes that accompany the HypnoVision program, please write to her in care of Clarity Unlimited, P.O. Box 540, Templeton, CA 93465.

Index

Oblique muscles (*cont'd*)
in myopia, 22–24, 173–74
in strabismus, 198, 200
Occipital lobe, 7
Optical center. *See* Brain
Optic nerve
dysfunctions of, 28
in normal vision, 14
Optometrists, xi, xiv, 1
on astigmatism, 185
attitude of, toward natural techniques, 5, 35
and floaters, 25
glaucoma checks by, 19
on lens accommodation, 11–12, 20–22
Ozone layer, 35

Palming, 45–46, 57–59, 132–33, 221
Pendulum technique, 51–52, 127–28, 171–72, 190, 195, 205–7, 219
Partner, working with. *See* HypnoVision program—with partner
Peripheral vision
glaucoma and, 19
retinal function in, 13
in retinitis pigmentosa, 27
Pineal gland, 13, 33
Ping-Pong, 228
"Pink eye" (conjunctivitis), 16, 30
Pituitary gland, 13, 33
Placebo effect, 37–38
Play, approaching "work" sessions as, 147, 148, 229
Positive suggestion, xiii. *See also* Hypnotherapy; HypnoVision program
Postural Integration, 32
Posture, xii, 18, 32, 186
Presbyopia, 1, 6, 129–72
age and, 20, 129–31
diet and, 130, 131, 172
exercise and, 130, 131, 172
HypnoVision program for, 132–72
accommodation exercise, 147, 153–60
evaluating need for further work, 171–72

induction, 132, 133, *see also* Induction
maintenance sessions, 130
massages, 136–46
minisessions, 131, 132, 135, 137, 141–42
palming, 132–33
reading skills, 160–71
scheduling, 131
string fusion, 147–53, 160
iris and pupil in, 20
smoking and, 21, 130
vitamins and, 31, 130
Psychoanalysis, 40
Pupil
in myopia, 20
in normal vision, 9–10
in presbyopia, 20

Rachmaninoff, Sergei, 54–55
Radiation
from computer screens, 33, 34
from fluorescent lighting, 33
Radix Institute, xii–xiii, 3, 174
Reading
and astigmatism, 18
hyperopia in children and, 174
nearpoint
for bifocal/trifocal wearers, 195
in hyperopia program, 183
in presbyopia program, 160–71
fever and, 29
lighting and, 33
Recti muscles. *See also* Vision exercises
in astigmatism, 185–90
definition of, 11
in hyperopia, 24, 173–74
in strabismus, 198–201
Regression technique, 26, 27, 127, 175, 185, 219–26
definition of, 220
emotional factors and, 219–20
with partner, 220
in strabismus, 196
instructions for, 220–25
Reich, Wilhelm, xiii, 24
Reincarnation, 225